Marketing to Pharmacists: Understanding Their Role and Influence

Marketing to Pharmacists: Understanding Their Role and Influence has been co-published simultaneously as *Journal of Pharmaceutical Marketing Practice*, Volume 1, Number 2 (#2) 1998.

Journal of Pharmaceutical Marketing Practice Monographic "Separates"

Below is a list of "separates," which in serials librarianship means a special issue simultaneously published as a special journal issue or double-issue and as a "separate" hardbound monograph. (This is a format which we also call a "Docuserial.")

"Separates" are published because specialized libraries or professionals may wish to purchase a specific thematic issue by itself in a format which can be separately cataloged and shelved, as opposed to purchasing the journal on an on-going basis. Faculty members may also more easily consider a "separate" for classroom adoption.

"Separates" are carefully classified separately with the major book jobbers so that the journal tie-in can be noted on new book order slips to avoid duplicate purchasing.

You may wish to visit the Haworth's website at . . .

http://www.haworthpressinc.com

. . . to search our online catalog for complete tables of contents of these separates and related publications.

You may also call 1-800-HAWORTH (outside US/Canada: 607-722-5857), or Fax 1-800-895-0582 (outside US/Canada: 607-771-0012), or e-mail at:

getinfo@haworthpressinc.com

Marketing to Pharmacists: Understanding Their Role and Influence

Marketing to Pharmacists: Understanding Their Role and Influence
has been co-published simultaneously as *Journal of Pharmaceutical
Marketing Practice*, Volume 1, Number 2 (#2) 1998.

Benjamin F. Banahan III, Ph.D.
Editor

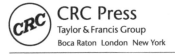

CRC Press
Taylor & Francis Group
Boca Raton London New York

CRC Press is an imprint of the
Taylor & Francis Group, an **informa** business

CRC Press
Taylor & Francis Group
6000 Broken Sound Parkway NW, Suite 300
Boca Raton, FL 33487-2742

© 1998 by Taylor & Francis Group, LLC
CRC Press is an imprint of Taylor & Francis Group, an Informa business

No claim to original U.S. Government works

Visit the Taylor & Francis Web site at
http://www.taylorandfrancis.com

and the CRC Press Web site at
http://www.crcpress.com

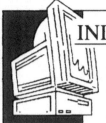

Marketing to Pharmacists: Understanding Their Role and Influence

CONTENTS

ABOUT THE EDITOR

Benjamin F. Banahan III, Ph.D., is a Research Professor and Coordinator of the Pharmaceutical Marketing and Management Research Program in the Research Institute of Pharmaceutical Sciences and Professor of Pharmacy Administration in the School of Pharmacy at the University of Mississippi. He received a B.S. in Psychology from Louisiana State University and a M.S. and Ph.D. in Health Care Administration from the University of Mississippi. Prior to assuming his current position at the University of Mississippi, Dr. Banahan was on the faculty at the School of Primary Medical Care at the University of Alabama in Huntsville.

Dr. Banahan has authored or coauthored more than 70 publications appearing in professional journals and magazines. He has also been an author on more than 160 peer-reviewed and invited papers presented at professional association and scientific meetings. Dr. Banahan is very active in continuing education activities, conducting numerous seminars and workshops each year for health care professionals and/or marketing research practitioners working in the pharmaceutical industry. He is actively involved in conducting primary research. His major research interests include generic substitution, therapeutic recommendations and interchange, managed care formulary trends, and pharmaceutical pricing.

Introduction

Benjamin F. Banahan III
Lisa A. Basara

The pharmaceutical marketplace has changed considerably during the last decade. Managed care is the predominant form of third-party coverage, and cost containment is a key goal for all members of the health care system. Among prescription product benefits, patient outcomes and cost-effectiveness now rank as highly as safety and efficacy. Patients have also joined the list of key customers for the pharmaceutical industry. Patients are more involved in their care; they assume direct responsibility and actively participate in therapy-related decisions. The increasing popularity of direct-to-consumer advertising (DTCA), Internet-based health information sites, and consumer-oriented medication references books are just some signs of this phenomenon. For pharmaceutical marketers and market researchers, this changing marketplace has resulted in more (and more complex) customers, each with diverse needs and desires. It remains critical for pharmaceutical marketers and market researchers to understand, assess, and respond to the needs of these customers, as well as those of physicians, nurses, and other traditional marketing targets.

Benjamin F. Banahan III, Ph.D., is Research Professor and Coordinator for the Pharmaceutical Marketing and Management Research Program, Waller Lab Complex, Research Institute of Pharmaceutical Sciences, and Professor of Pharmacy Administration, School of Pharmacy, University of Mississippi, University, MS 38677. E-mail: ribfb@olemiss.edu

Lisa A. Basara, Ph.D., is a consultant with The Resolutions Group, 4000 Skippack Pike, 2nd Floor, Skippack, PA 19474.

[Haworth co-indexing entry note]: "Introduction." Banahan, Benjamin F., III, and Lisa A. Basara. Co-published simultaneously in *Journal of Pharmaceutical Marketing Practice* (Pharmaceutical Products Press, an imprint of The Haworth Press, Inc.) Vol. 1, No. 2 (#2), 1998, pp. 1-2; and: *Marketing to Pharmacists: Understanding Their Role and Influence* (ed: Benjamin F. Banahan III) Pharmaceutical Products Press, an imprint of The Haworth Press, Inc., 1998, pp. 1-2. Single or multiple copies of this article are available for a fee from The Haworth Document Delivery Service [1-800-342-9678, 9:00 a.m. - 5:00 p.m. (EST). E-mail address: getinfo@haworthpressinc.com].

The last decade has also challenged community pharmacists to understand, assess, and respond to changes in the pharmaceutical marketplace. Computers and robotics have usurped the dispensing process, threatening a primary function of community pharmacists. However, while these technologies are a potential threat, they also give pharmacists an opportunity to monitor drug therapies and to provide comprehensive patient care. As evidence of this professional struggle, dominant topics at recent state and national pharmacy meetings have included defining pharmaceutical care and identifying community pharmacy's role in patient care management.

This collection of articles examines important trends in pharmaceutical health care, including patient education and compliance, quality of life assessment, disease management, and cost-containment strategies. A common link among all of these trends is community pharmacy. Pharmacists in both retail and independently owned stores influence prescription product selection, monitor drug therapy, and serve as a primary source of patient education.

As a key customer of the pharmaceutical industry, pharmaceutical marketers and market researchers must understand the role of and issues that affect community pharmacy. This collection is a comprehensive resource about community pharmacists and the trends that they influence.

A History Lesson:
Can You Dispense with Pharmacists?

Editor's Note: "Can You Dispense with Pharmacists?" was first published in 1974. It is being reprinted as part of this collection for at least two reasons. First, the article helps us to appreciate that even when it appears that rapid and dramatic change is imminent, change seldom occurs as rapidly or dramatically as we think it will. For those of us who can remember what was going on in 1974, the health care system was in a state of crisis, cost containment concerns were going to change everything, and independent pharmacies were doomed to be extinct within a few years. Today we can see that some changes have occurred in the health care system, but the changes have not been as dramatic as predicted in the mid 1970's. In fact, many of the same problems and impending changes are still looming over us.

The second reason for reprinting this article is that it described how the pharmacist-industry relationship had shifted from one of partnership to one of adversaries and issued a call for pharmaceutical marketers to develop a better understanding of pharmacists so both groups could realize the potential partnership that could exist. Unfortunately, the pharmacist-industry relationship is probably more strained today than it was in 1974. However, the other articles in this collection can help pharmaceutical marketers better understand what is occurring in pharmaceutical practice today, and they identify a variety of ways in

Mickey C. Smith, Ph.D., is F.A.P. Barnard Distinguished Professor of Pharmacy Administration at the University of Mississippi School of Pharmacy, University, MS 38677.

Presented to the Pharmaceutical Advertising Club of Montreal, Canada, February 19, 1974.

This article was first published in *Medical Marketing and Media* in June 1974 (pp. 28-31) and is reprinted with permission.

[Haworth co-indexing entry note]: "A History Lesson: Can You Dispense with Pharmacists?" Smith, Mickey C. Co-published simultaneously in *Journal of Pharmaceutical Marketing Practice* (Pharmaceutical Products Press, an imprint of The Haworth Press, Inc.) Vol. 1, No. 2 (#2), 1998, pp. 3-10; and: *Marketing to Pharmacists: Understanding Their Role and Influence* (ed: Benjamin F. Banahan III) Pharmaceutical Products Press, an imprint of The Haworth Press, Inc., 1998, pp. 3-10.

3

which pharmaceutical marketers can develop better relationships with pharmacists in community practice.

The idea for the title of this article came to me while reading an issue of *Pharmacy Times* magazine, in which appeared a cartoon showing the interior of a pharmacy with the slogan over the prescription department reading *"We dispense with accuracy."* As I pondered the two possible meanings of that slogan, I developed the rhetorical question which now serves as the topic of my presentation–can you dispense with pharmacists? Can you do *without* them? Or what can you do *with* them?

Who *is* the pharmacist anyway?

In fact, there are many pharmacists–many types, many kinds–filled with conflicting motivations, conflicting desires, and practicing in a variety of settings and under diverse working conditions. Yet, in spite of this, as working men and women, your job, as I understand it, is to identify the pharmacist as a marketing target and perhaps as a marketing partner. How can this be done?

While the corner drug store is a common enough establishment, sociologically speaking, pharmacy is a most unusual occupation. It has been described as a profession in search of an occupation. It has also been described as the most overtrained or underutilized of the health professions. Back in 1955, a Canadian sociologist, Thelma Herman McCormick, first coined the term "marginal profession" to describe pharmacy (I won't comment on the appropriateness of someone with two names such as Thelma and Herman calling someone else marginal). By marginal professional she meant a group of people who, as she determined from her study, were uncertain whether they were professional people or businessmen (it is not important today to determine or to discuss whether the two are incompatible).

Her phrase has been quoted time and time again since that study was completed, and there seems little evidence today that there has been much change in the "marginality" of pharmacy, at least at the retail drug store level.

We have, then, a person who has in most cases a college education (and in many cases five years of a college education), designed to train him to practice pharmacy; a person who has been told throughout his pharmacy training that he is a professional; who has received from his pharmacy educators an almost constant barrage of caveats concerning the horrors of "merchandising" and the dangers of too much involvement with the "front end" of the drug store.

Here is a person who may have been (in fact probably was) attracted to pharmacy in the first place because of what he could *see* in the retail drug business, who in his pharmacy education was told that most of these things were the wrong reasons for entering pharmacy school, and who (if he is typical) upon graduation was told by his employer that all the professors were lost in their ivory towers and that the *business* end of the drug store was where the action was. Now this pharmacist is *really* confused. He doesn't know who he is, or who he's supposed to be, nor what to do to change his way of life to fit his personal needs as well as the needs of his clients. And you folks haven't *helped* any either.

The messages he receives from the pharmaceutical industry have been just as confusing. Advertising to pharmacists runs the gamut from the purely professional (*"You're the last stop in the process of drug therapy; Your opinion is important in regard to drugs; We need you,"* etc.) to the totally and blatantly commercial message (*Stock up now, there'll be lots of profits and lots of dollars if you buy plenty of our product and push it hard*).

The fact is, you don't seem to know who the pharmacist is either. I have been told by one advertising executive that the pharmacist is becoming more important. He still can't do the manufacturer any good, but he can do him real harm. I guess that's progress of sorts.

Let's get back to our original question–can you dispense with pharmacists? Let's take the first meaning. Can you get along without them? I believe personally that the answer to that question would have to be *"No."* Given the current health care system, the pharmaceutical industry is dependent for its distribution on the pharmacist (or someone yet to be developed like the pharmacist). Because of the current legal restrictions on drug distribution, someone called a pharmacist must be involved in the distribution of prescription drugs. Because of the social tradition of the drug store someone like a pharmacist is probably going to be involved in the distribution of nonprescription drugs (even though I will admit that vast quantities of nonprescription drugs are being distributed without ever being touched or perhaps even being seen by a pharmacist).

The pharmacist's importance to you as marketers seems likely to be enhanced by increasing generic prescribing, whether such prescribing results from Government fiat or simply because more and more physicians become accustomed to this practice and motivated to it for whatever their reasons.

With this in mind, I would have to give a qualified *"no"* to the question of whether pharmacists can be done away with as a marketing partner. So let's move on to the second part of that question. Can you (the pharmaceutical marketer) work with the pharmacist in the dispensing process? Or putting it another way: can you develop a partnership with the pharmacist in all phases of the marketing of prescription and nonprescription drugs? The answer to that question is an easy one, and it is of course, *"yes."* The pharmaceutical industry is already working with the pharmacist. He is dispensing their drugs, stocking their drugs, filling prescriptions with their drugs. But a further question might be, *"Can we do it better, and if so, how?"* My position on this would be that in order for pharmaceutical marketers to realize the fullest potential of the partnership between manufacturer and pharmacist will require a much better understanding of the pharmacist by those who must market to him and through him.

Let's talk about some specifics, and let's begin with the pronoun I used in my previous sentence. The pronoun was "him." I could say that I intentionally used that as a lead-in to my next point, but in fact like the rest of you, I tend to think of the pharmacist as a male. Now you may be getting a bit tired of hearing about women's liberation, but as marketing people I am sure you are aware that sex does occasionally rear its provocative head. Within pharmacy circles, any trend line you tend to draw would lead to the inescapable conclusion that females are now a major factor in pharmacy and, further, that their influence and contribution to pharmacy is going to increase rapidly. The proportion of females in pharmacy schools in Canada is approaching or perhaps has already surpassed 40 percent. In the United States it's 25 percent, but it was 10 percent just 15 years ago.

Some of the ramifications of this are fairly obvious. For example, females are going to have to start appearing in your advertising to pharmacists. Are you doing this or have you given it any thought?

Some of the more subtle concerns, however, should also figure in your planning. Females generally, in spite of anything you may have heard to the contrary, are different from males. Their goals are different, their orientation toward such things as merchandising and management is different, their work pattern differs, and the things which motivate them differ.

Most female pharmacists are employees. There are proportionately few female pharmacy owners. Many female pharmacists are not the primary wage earner in the family and thus (although their salaries are important) the livelihood of their families may not depend on their individual earnings. For these reasons, marketing to female pharmacists will probably have to take on a considerably different character than has been the pattern in the past.

You are going to have some new partners in the future and perhaps the majority will be female.

Speaking of partners, what has happened to the old partnership which used to characterize the pharmacist-industry relationship? When Senator Kefauver was having his field day in this country, organized pharmacy and organized industry followed pretty much the same line in answering his charges. They were together in this fight. Now that Senator Nelson and of course Senator Kennedy are engaged in the same general kind of investigation, pharmacy and industry seem to be miles apart. What has happened? Well, of course, we'll never know all the answers to this, but let's consider a couple of items.

The first thing I would like you to ponder should involve some pretty heavy sociological study which I have not given it, and which would probably not be too interesting to you anyway. But consider for the moment the fact that the art of pharmacy was taken over by the pharmaceutical industry some twenty or so years ago. The mystery of compounding and the exotic smells and sounds of the prescription department have largely disappeared because the pharmaceutical industry has turned into a mass production process. We all know the benefits which accrued to the public (and to pharmacy as well) by these changes, but the fact remains that the art of pharmacy as it *used* to exist is gone and that the drug industry took it.

Now I don't know to what extent the pharmacist has formally considered this, but I do know that the industry gave him nothing to hang onto in return. Literally, ever since the 1950's when the real pharmaceutical revolution really took hold, pharmacy has been casting about for other things on which to hang its hat. One of these is the so-called expert "drug consultant" label. Industry has not promoted this possibility for reasons which I am sure are compelling to them. They have fought on the generic issue for obvious reasons and have not encouraged their patients to consult with the pharmacist on non-prescription drugs. (The current Burroughs-Wellcome campaign is a welcome exception.) So, in essence, they have given the pharmacist very little in return for what they have taken away.

At a meeting held in the early part of 1974, when organized pharmacy was fighting for recognition by the FDA of the role of the pharmacist as a consultant on nonprescription drugs, what was the position of industry? The chairman of Miles Laboratories testified:

> *"I see no real need for professional intervention between the label and the user. If there is, it shouldn't be an OTC product in the first place."*

I believe that the pharmacist may not see the industry as his partner any more, but rather as some sort of adversary. This is a tragedy when one considers that, whatever else the pharmacist's hangups may be, he could and should enjoy a positive marketing image in the eyes of the manufacturer.

The pharmacist *does* depend upon the manufacturer and the manufacturer *does* depend on the pharmacist. Yet, I know of no other industry (with the possible exception of the current situation in the gasoline business) where the manufacturer and the retailer are approaching an adversary position.

Another sociological consideration for you is the eternal triangle of physician, pharmacist, and manufacturer. When I was in pharmacy school we were taught that whatever the doctor says *goes*. This isn't what is being taught today. Many old pharmacists, being human, *resent* the old subservient role. Many feel, however, that there is little they can do about it. It is natural, however, for them to also resent the obvious difference in the amount of industry attention (and money) devoted to the doctor as compared to the pharmacist. Is it any wonder that there is a little natural satisfaction at the discomfort of the industry when it is faced with generics and substitution and suddenly the *pharmacist* becomes important?

Considerable time has been spent by pharmacists in looking for other things to do and other lines of endeavor in which to engage. There has been talk of using the pharmacist in high blood pressure monitoring and education, using the pharmacist as an intermediary in family planning, using the pharmacist as a health food expert. Indeed there has been a variety of new roles and new activities postulated for pharmacists. The industry has been strangely silent in these discussions.

Well, not completely silent–perhaps just a little myopic. Back in October, John Horan, senior vice-president of Merck & Company, Inc., addressed the National Association of Retail Druggists under a title of "An Undermedicated Society." His message cited *"large numbers of Americans who fail to receive prescription drugs which could protect their health and life."* And he was right to do so. The examples he used (hypertension, diabetes, arthritis, depression, venereal disease) are all areas in which pharmacy has shown evidence of seeking new responsibilities.

Now here, it seems to me, is an opportunity which, if seized, results in benefits for all. The public gets the drugs it needs, the pharmacists get some new responsibilities, and the manufacturers sales increase. Here is a chance for the manufacturer to help pharmacy innovate in the delivery of expanded services in the primary care, diagnostic, and preventive medicine areas. Here is where all of that high powered marketing know-how and imagination can find an application which might result in benefits for all concerned.

Yet we haven't seen much of that. Why not? For one thing the physician can be expected to raise hell. Mr. Horan, if I understand him, can only recommend a sort of glorified public relations campaign. (If I'm wrong, and he's ready for something stronger, I'm all for him.) And that's not the answer to anybody's problems now.

Perhaps the industry isn't sure of the validity of these new ideas, but I wonder if you are overlooking some potential marketing possibilities. Pharmacy has demonstrated itself as an effective (if not necessarily efficient) retail operation. New activities for the pharmacist should mean new marketing opportunities for the industry. What have you done to explore these possibilities? What have you done to encourage them as far as the pharmacist is concerned? I believe this is an area which deserves further investigation by informed marketing people.

In a small study in which we are presently conducting, more than one-half of the pharmacist respondents indicated that they would not choose pharmacy again if they had it to do over. This is the *frustration* expressing itself. Sometimes the future is expressed in *determination*. Listen to Eugene White.

> *"I am saying opportunity is knocking at the door of the private practitioner; this is commencement for us! Will contemporary retail pharmacy survive? No! Will private practice survive? I say yes! We are alive, healthy, and kicking vigorously! When the prescription order no longer crosses your threshold but originates in your office at the tip of your pen, think of the impact on all facets of health care: the health care team, the Government, the Drug Enforcement Administration, the FDA, the pharmaceutical industry, the chains and mail-order operations, the insurance carriers, the national health programs, and most of all–your patient.*
>
> *"Emerson said, 'Every revolution was first a thought in one man's mind, and when the same thought occurs to another man, it is the key to that era.' I'm no Emerson, but by God, I can read the road signs. Dissatisfaction, unhappiness, restlessness, impatience makes one search for something new–something better. If this kind of restlessness produces dissent and disturbs the respectable and comfortable status quo, so be it!"*

Now how are you betting on the future of pharmacy? How do your actions reflect your bet? What are you doing to get to know the pharmacist? Are you checking both sides of this marginal personality? Have you concerned yourself only with the pharmacist as a marketing man and ignored the professionalization process which pharmacy is going through?

To those who are not pharmacists, I suggest that they make an effort to get to know pharmacists at the practice level. We feel so strongly about this at the University of Mississippi that we are putting together a special five-day intensive course in marketing to pharmacists. This will involve a complete immersion by a limited number of marketing people in the pharmacy environment. They will get to meet and spend time with pharmacists practicing in a variety of settings, they will attend classes with pharmacy students, participate in roundtable discussion, shop for prescription and nonprescription drugs, and do a variety of things which we believe will eventually result in a much deeper understanding of the pharmacist as a marketing partner, marketing target, and human being.

Community Pharmacists' Influence on Prescription Drug Choices

Benjamin F. Banahan III

INTRODUCTION

When asked what the pharmacist's role in the prescription product selection is, many pharmaceutical marketers would respond, "Deciding whether to use a generic or not." People who have had experience with programs designed to reward product switching, especially if their company was not the one promoting the switch campaign, might respond, "Performing generic and therapeutic substitution."

In examining the role of community pharmacists in prescription product selection, the first response definitely is too narrow and in many ways is like describing what you see when looking at an iceberg: it addresses the most visible and talked about behavior, but only represents a small portion of the overall role pharmacists play in product selection. Although generic substitution receives considerable attention in the professional and lay press, it is only one of several ways in which community pharmacists have an impact on prescription product selection. The second response adds another potential role to the list, but it is an emotional overstatement and in almost every situation is

Benjamin F. Banahan III, Ph.D., is Research Professor and Coordinator for the Pharmaceutical Marketing and Management Research Program, Waller Lab Complex, Research Institute of Pharmaceutical Sciences, and Professor of Pharmacy Administration, School of Pharmacy, University of Mississippi, University, MS 38677. E-mail: ribfb@olemiss.edu

[Haworth co-indexing entry note]: "Community Pharmacists' Influence on Prescription Drug Choices." Banahan, Benjamin F., III. Co-published simultaneously in *Journal of Pharmaceutical Marketing Practice* (Pharmaceutical Products Press, an imprint of The Haworth Press, Inc.) Vol. 1, No. 2 (#2), 1998, pp. 11-35; and: *Marketing to Pharmacists: Understanding Their Role and Influence* (ed: Benjamin F. Banahan III) Pharmaceutical Products Press, an imprint of The Haworth Press, Inc., 1998, pp. 11-35. Single or multiple copies of this article are available for a fee from The Haworth Document Delivery Service [1-800-342-9678, 9:00 a.m. - 5:00 p.m. (EST). E-mail address: getinfo@haworthpressinc.com].

technically an incorrect description of another way that pharmacists frequently do influence prescription product selection.

The role of the community pharmacist in prescription product selection has evolved over the last three decades and may be changing more rapidly today than at any time in the history of pharmaceuticals. When people in the pharmaceutical industry perceive the role of community pharmacists in prescription product selection as being described by one of the simple responses given above, they seriously underestimate the influence these practitioners have and usually develop marketing strategies that do not appropriately address the true process of product selection in community pharmacy practice today.

The objectives of this article are to overcome some of the limitations of these two typical responses by defining and pointing out the differences between some of pharmacists' behaviors related to product selection; to document, when possible, the extent to which each behavior influences product selection; and to provide pharmaceutical marketers with a better understanding of how community pharmacists influence product selection so companies can develop more effective marketing strategies.

IMPORTANT TERMINOLOGY

Unfortunately, the terms used to describe the activities of pharmacists that influence which drug product actually is dispensed to a patient are inconsistent among publications, presentations, and reports produced by and for health professionals, the public, and the pharmaceutical industry. The confusion has become a more serious problem as managed care organizations and pharmaceutical manufacturers have become actively involved in attempts to encourage or discourage pharmacists from influencing the product selection process. The misuse of terms has often resulted in what appear to be gross overstatements of the prevalence of certain behaviors and a misunderstanding of the actual process involved in almost all of these activities.

Perhaps one of the best examples of how the inconsistent and/or inappropriate use of terms can result in poor professional relations and misunderstandings between pharmacists and manufacturers has been the misuse of the terms "therapeutic interchange" and "therapeutic substitution." These terms have often been used to describe the therapeutic recommendations pharmacists make to patients and prescribers which result in prescriptions being changed from one product to an alternative therapeutic agent. As described below, therapeutic recommendations of this nature are very different from the process of therapeutic interchange which typically occurs only in institutional settings. Community pharmacists performing therapeutic recommendations do not consider themselves to be performing, and are not performing, "therapeutic substitution." When this term is applied to the act of making a therapeutic recommendation, it results in an overstatement of the frequency of therapeutic substitution and often results in serious miscommunication. Hopefully the following definitions will assist in pointing out the sometimes subtle, but nonetheless important, distinctions among generic substitution, therapeutic substitution or interchange, and therapeutic recommendations.

Generic substitution (or interchange) is the dispensing of a bioequivalent generic drug product for a prescription written for a brand-name drug product without contacting the prescriber. Which products can be substituted, whether pharmacists "must" or "may" substitute, and the manner in which prescribers can restrict generic substitution are identified in the pharmacy practice acts and regulations of each state. Within the pharmacy literature and in many state regulations, generic substitution is often referred to as "product selection." The history of generic substitution regulations and trends in generic substitution behaviors are discussed in more detail in the following section.

It is important to note that, according to the technical definition of generic substitution, a pharmacist only performs generic substitution when a prescription is written for or has previously been filled with one manufacturer's product (i.e., the brand-name product) and the pharmacist, using his/her professional judgment, decides to dispense a therapeutically equivalent and generically equivalent product manufactured by a different company, *without* consultation with the prescriber. Generic substitution occurs when switches are made between a brand product and a generic, as well as when changes are made from one generic manufacturer to another.

A key element in this definition is that the change in manufacturers occurs without prescriber consultation. When pharmacists contact the prescriber and discuss the possibility of switching manufacturers, they have not performed generic substitution. In this case, they are making a therapeutic recommendation–the use of a different manufacturer-

and when the prescriber agrees to accept the recommendation, the prescription has technically been modified over the phone to be a prescription written for the recommended product.

Another potential issue that causes some confusion with respect to generic substitution is the terminology used by the FDA in classifying the acceptability of products for interchange. The FDA uses the term "therapeutic equivalents" to define pharmaceutically equivalent products (products that contain the same active ingredients and are identical in strength, concentration, dosage form, and route of administration) that are expected to have the same therapeutic effect based on their having been determined to be bioequivalent (1). With the increase in therapeutic substitution that has occurred during the last decade, the terms "generic equivalents" and "therapeutic equivalents" have often been used to describe products that could be generically substituted and therapeutically substituted, respectively. This more limited use of the term "therapeutic equivalent" can cause confusion when it is not distinguished from the way the term is used by the FDA.

Therapeutic substitution (or *interchange*) is the dispensing of a therapeutically equivalent but generically inequivalent drug without contacting the prescriber for permission at the time of dispensing. Again, it is important to note that a key part of the definition is that the substitution of products occurs without notification of or consultation with the prescriber at the time that the alternative product is dispensed.

When allowed by state practice regulations, therapeutic substitution is performed by having prescribers and pharmacists agree in advance on protocols and/or formulary guidelines that stipulate when and what substitutions will be allowed. Therapeutic substitution is accomplished in most institutional settings, such as hospitals and HMOs, by having a Pharmacy and Therapeutics (P&T) Committee develop a formulary identifying preferred products considered to be therapeutically equivalent in treating certain conditions. Physicians practicing within the institution are required to review the formulary and to sign an agreement that therapeutic substitution can be performed according to the formulary. When a physician prescribes a product other than the preferred product, the substitution is made and notation is made in the patient's chart; in some settings, a notification is sent to the prescribing physician. As with generic substitution, the fact that the product change is made without contacting the prescriber before each occurrence is the characteristic that makes this a therapeutic substitution rather than a therapeutic recommendation.

Although therapeutic substitution occurs in the majority of hospitals, it typically will be performed only for a small number of products (2). Because therapeutic substitution requires prior consent by the prescriber and a well-defined protocol for substitution, therapeutic substitution is seldom performed outside of institutions such as hospitals, staff-model HMOs, etc. Since a therapeutic substitution protocol is the ultimate in formulary control of product selection, it is not surprising that pharmaceutical manufacturers have expressed serious concerns about the widespread application of therapeutic substitution (3).

Therapeutic recommendation is a professional suggestion made to a patient and/or the prescriber that a change be made in a prescription. Therapeutic recommendations have always been an important part of the product selection process, providing a checks-and-balances system to guard against inappropriate prescribing, potential drug interactions, etc. During the last decade, therapeutic recommendations have become an even more important part of the product selection process, going beyond the original checks-and-balances aspect to play a more active role in therapy management.

In contrast to generic and therapeutic substitution, contact and consultation with the prescriber prior to dispensing an alternative product *does* occur with therapeutic recommendation. This consultation is the essence of a therapeutic recommendation. The basic premise of therapeutic recommendations is that the pharmacist is making a professional recommendation that a change be made in a prescription. If the recommendation is not accepted, the prescription will stand as received by the pharmacist and will be dispensed accordingly. When the recommendation is accepted by the prescriber, the original prescription is actually replaced by a new medication order or prescription that has been communicated to the pharmacist verbally during the conversation. In such a situation, the pharmacist has not substituted an alternative product; instead, the prescriber has opted to change the prescription in response to a professional recommendation.

Although some of the distinction between therapeutic substitution and therapeutic recommendation may appear to be simply semantics, the distinction is a very serious one with respect to pharmacy law and regulations. In most states, therapeutic substitution can only be done within institutional settings and even then under rather limited circumstances. Some states do allow for therapeutic substitution to be performed in community practice under written protocol agreed to by the prescriber. Regardless of the setting, therapeutic substitution requires prior written approval be obtained from the prescriber, while generic substitution does not require any prior approval. Therapeutic recommendations, on the other hand, can and are done in almost every pharmacy setting and are one of the major ways in which formularies are enforced in hospitals and other institutional settings. Therapeutic recommendations also can address a much broader array of therapeutic issues than generic or therapeutic substitution can. Therapeutic recommendations can include suggestions regarding changes in dosing, switching to alternative products, adding additional drug therapies, changing to alternative nonpharmacological treatment options, etc.

GENERIC SUBSTITUTION

Generic substitution has increased considerably during the last decade. This rapid increase is the result of a variety of changes that have occurred in our health care environment. To better understand the rise in the use of generics and the forces that are encouraging this increased use, it is necessary to review some of the history of generics in the United States.

The original state antisubstitution laws were not passed to prevent the use of the legally approved generics we have today. During the 1950's, compounding was very common, and counterfeiting of prescription drugs had become a serious problem. The American Pharmaceutical Association (APhA) and the Pharmaceutical Manufacturers Association (PMA) joined together to promote the establishment of antisubstitution laws in the states to control drug counterfeiting. Cooperative action among the pharmaceutical associations, the state boards of pharmacy, and the pharmaceutical manufacturers led to the adoption of laws and/or regulations forbidding substitution in almost every state (4).

The political playing field did not change much with respect to substitution until health care costs became an increasingly popular political issue and drug approval regulations were developed that resulted in the marketing of "approved" generic drug products. In 1962, the Kefauver-Harris Drug Amendment was passed. The amendment required that a drug awaiting approval had to show efficacy in addition to safety and changed the definition of the term "new drug" to mean the "entire dosage form" instead of just the "therapeutic chemical entity" (5). A major result of this legislation was that generic drugs had to file full NDAs to be approved for marketing. Obviously, this regulation greatly restricted the introduction of generic drugs.

As would be expected, with an NDA being required and antisubstitution legislation in place in almost every state, generic drugs represented a very limited market during the 1960's. However, in the 1970's, things began to change. In 1970, the FDA approved the abbreviated new drug application (ANDA) procedure for use with products approved for marketing between 1938 and 1962. The ANDA process greatly reduced the cost of obtaining approval of generic drugs and opened the door for the growth of the generic drug industry.

Also in 1970, the APhA reversed its stand of the previous 15-20 years and committed itself to seek the repeal of antisubstitution laws (4). Its position had not really changed, but the nature of substitution had shifted from the substitution of counterfeit products to the substitution of legitimate generically equivalent products. At the time, APhA defined substitution as the "substitution of one manufacturer's therapeutically effective and chemically equivalent drug product for the product of another prescribed by brand name alone." The APhA definition excluded counterfeit drugs and "secret remedies," which were the focus of the association's opposition to substitution 20 years earlier. The new stand by APhA was vehemently opposed by the PMA, which argued that the choice of drug and manufacturer should be reserved for the physician.

Perhaps the two events that had the greatest effect on establishing the current trend in generic drug use in America are the FDA's approval of the ANDA procedure in 1970 and establishment by the Department of Health and Human Services of maximum allowable costs (MACs) for reimbursement of selected generic drugs under Medicaid. The introduction of ANDAs greatly reduced the cost and time required for obtaining approval of generics, thus making it possible for a relatively large number of companies to more easily enter and compete in the generic pharmaceutical market. Although the ANDA process created the possibility of a highly competitive generic market, many states still had antisubstitution laws on the books that had been designed to prevent counterfeiting. When the MAC program was adopted in 1975, it became impossible for states with antisubstitution laws to participate in the Medicaid program because the cost of brand-name products was frequently greater than the MAC (5). The MAC program quickly led to the elimination of antisubstitution laws and, in many cases, resulted in new generic substitution regulations that actually encouraged the use of generics.

Another major boost to the generic industry occurred in 1984 with the passage of the Drug Price Competition and Patent Term Restoration Act. This act extended the ANDA procedure to drugs approved for marketing after 1962, making generic competition possible for many of the newer block buster products. It also allowed generic companies to begin bioequivalency studies before patent expiration which resulted in more generic companies entering the market immediately after patent launch, thus eroding the brand market even faster. Since 1980, the increasing number of products losing patent protection, the relaxing of regulatory barriers to generics, and the growing pressure for health care cost control has resulted in a rapid growth of the generic drug industry.

Although pharmacists in the late 1970's saw an increase in pressures to dispense generics, there were many concerns that limited the initial use of generics (6, 7). An early problem was the difficulty pharmacists had in determining which products were acceptable substitutes. Through the encouragement of state Medicaid agencies, in 1980 the FDA began publication of the *Approved Drug Products with Therapeutic Equivalence Evaluations*, which is commonly referred to as the *Orange Book*. With the publication of the *Orange Book*, pharmacists had an easy way to determine which products could be substituted.

As generic drug use slowly became more acceptable and prevalent during the late 1970's and early 1980's, the rate of generic penetration became somewhat predictable for most products. During the late 1980's, many manufacturers adopted regular price increases as their primary strategy to compensate for the market share they knew they would lose to generics. This, coupled with the rising average price of prescription products, led to significant increases in the political, economic, and patient forces encouraging the use of generics in community pharmacy.

Patient Price Sensitivity

Community pharmacy has often been referred to as the last three feet of the pharmaceutical distribution system. This is an accurate description in that the community pharmacy is where the physical product literally reaches the hands of the patient. The close personal nature of this transfer of product from the pharmacist to the patient or the patient's representative is important in that it presents an opportunity for interaction between the patient and provider that can result in better patient care (i.e., patient counseling). It also provides an opportunity for the patient to become more involved in his or her care and, to some degree, the selection of the product that will be dispensed. During the last few decades, patients have become increasingly involved in product selection by asking for generics, questioning prices, and asking about or requesting specific prescription products they have seen advertised.

One of the major factors leading to the increase in patient inquiries about generics is the commonly promoted image that generics are less expensive. Two surveys conducted by the University of Mississippi found that pharmacists' estimates of the percentage of their patients inquiring about lower cost therapies increased from 30% in 1990 to 38% in 1992 (8, 9). Similar increases in patients requesting generics have been reported in other surveys. Surveys conducted by *Drug Topics* found that from 1991 to 1994 the percentage of pharmacists who said patients frequently request generics increased from 47% to 59% (10). In the 1994 *Drug Topics* survey, 91% of community pharmacists reported that their customers respond favorably to a pharmacist's suggestion that customers request generic prescriptions from their physicians.

Price Differentials and Profit Margins

By far, economic incentives have been–and still are–the major force driving the use of generics. There were senate hearings about the monopoly of the pharmaceutical industry throughout the 1960's, and "in 1966, the Task Force on Prescription Drugs recommended generic prescribing of drugs, and projected a wholesale cost savings of $41 million if 63 products were prescribed exclusively by generic names" (11). During the late 1980's, Senator Pryor conducted hearings about prescription drug costs, and once again, there were calls for the widespread use of generics as a means of saving health care dollars.

During the late 1970's and throughout the 1980's, the average prescription price began to rise rapidly. This probably was the result of

two major factors: the more aggressive, higher pricing of new innovative therapies and the frequent increases in prices of existing products.
The frequent price increases on existing products, especially those
with generic competition, have been identified as one of the major
strategies of pharmaceutical manufacturers for dealing with generic
competition during the 1980's. The pricing trends of the 1980's resulted in a rapid increase in patient and payer price sensitivity and
increased potential for profits for community pharmacy.

In a study conducted by the University of Mississippi in 1991,
pharmacists reported that a 32% price difference between the brand
and the generic was needed for them to consider substitution worthwhile and that they believed a 29% difference was needed for patients
to consider it worth substituting (12). In the same study, physicians
reported that a 32% price difference was needed for them to consider
substitution worthwhile and that only a 23% difference was needed for
patients to consider it worthwhile.

When brand manufacturers raised their prices in response to generic
erosion of their markets and generic manufacturers became increasingly competitive on price, the differentials between brand acquisition
costs and generic acquisition costs became greater. The size of this
cost differential provided community pharmacies an opportunity to
provide patients an adequate price savings (typically 30-50%) to address their perceptions of patients' price sensitivity while still pricing
generics in such a way as to increase their profit margin, especially in
the cash market, which up until just recently has made up the majority
of community pharmacy customers.

The examples in Table 1 show actual cost and retail price informa-

TABLE 1. Examples of Generic Product Profitability.				
	Acquisition Cost	Retail Price	Dollar Net Profit	% ROI
Naprosyn 500mg naproxen 500mg	$1.06 $0.15	$1.33 $0.73	$0.27 $0.58	25% 387%
Keftab© 500mg cephalexen 500mg	$1.69 $0.20	$2.41 $0.79	$0.72 $0.59	43% 295%

Source: Price-Chek. (Medi-Span, 1995)

tion for two products with generic alternatives. This information demonstrates how the cost differential between the brand and generic can be great enough to provide a very appealing situation for community pharmacists. When the generic market is highly competitive, the acquisition cost for the generic can be very low compared to the brand. The retail price is often set based on the perceived price sensitivity and market volume for each specific product. As shown in Table 1, the average retail price for naproxen 500mg provided patients with a 45% savings compared to the brand price while generating slightly more than twice the dollar net profit per tablet for pharmacies. When the retail price is set at a more competitive level, as demonstrated by cephalexen, patients received an average 67% savings, and although the pharmacies received slightly less dollar net profit per tablet, they still made an average 295% return on investment with the generic compared to an average 43% return on investment for the brand product. These examples illustrate how appealing generic prescription products can be for community pharmacies in that they provide the ultimate win-win situation where patients are provided a large savings compared to brand prices and the pharmacies' profits increase.

Store Policies and Managed Care Pressure

Store policies also can influence the degree to which pharmacists will promote generics in their day-to-day practice. A 1994 survey of community pharmacists conducted by the University of Mississippi found that 67% of community pharmacies had policies that encourage pharmacists to recommend generics to physicians and 87% of pharmacies have such policies to encourage the use of generics with customers (13). As shown in Figure 1, independent pharmacies were more likely than chain pharmacies to have such policies.

In addition to the direct financial incentive from net profits on cash sales, pharmacies also receive incentives from third parties to dispense generics. In a 1994 survey conducted by *Drug Topics*, 53% of pharmacists said they receive incentives to dispense generics (9). Increased dispensing fees were the most frequently cited form of incentive (41% of pharmacists), with other types of reimbursement incentives–such as cash rebates (12%) and higher reimbursement levels (11%)–also being mentioned.

FIGURE 1.   Percentage of Pharmacies Reporting Policies to Recommend
Generics to Physicians and Patients.

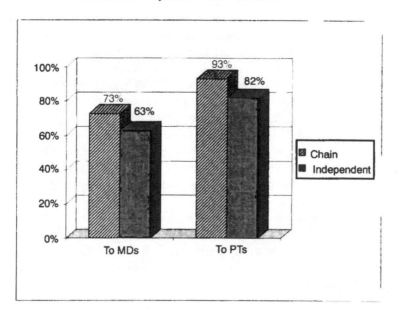

Source: Banahan BF III, Kolassa EM, McCaffrey DJ III. Generic substitution and narrow
therapeutic index drugs: a national survey of retail, hospital, managed care, and
nursing home pharmacists. University, MS: Research Institute of Pharmaceutical
Sciences, 1994.

Pharmacists' Attitudes Toward Generic Substitution

With each passing year since the first efforts to repeal the antisubstitution laws in the 1970's and 1980's, pharmacists and consumers
have become more accepting of generics. Even after the "generic
scandal" of 1989, consumer confidence in generics remained strong
and generic sales continued to increase at a rapid rate (14, 15). Pharmacists' attitudes toward substitution were examined frequently during
the 1970's and 1980's, when antisubstitution laws were being repealed
and generics were first being introduced into the market. Regular
surveys by *Drug Topics* and others have generally shown fairly strong
acceptance of generics, even following the 1989 scandal. Collectively,
pharmacists are fairly accepting of the therapeutic equivalency of
generic products and substitute without much concern. Although the

general acceptability of generics is not much of an issue today, the question of therapeutic equivalency for generics of narrow therapeutic index drugs has received considerable attention during the last few years.

In 1994, the University of Mississippi conducted a national survey that examined community pharmacists' attitudes toward substitution in general and substitution of critical dose drugs in particular (16). Overall, community pharmacists were found to agree fairly strongly with substitution in general, to perceive a fairly high level of influence encouraging them to substitute, and to be slightly concerned about substitution of critical dose drugs (Table 2). When pharmacists are segmented based on their attitudes, it becomes apparent that there are distinct subgroups of pharmacists who differ considerably with respect to these issues. Almost half of the pharmacists are in a cluster that is prosubstitution, heavily influenced to substitute, and moderately concerned about substitution of critical dose drugs. The remaining pharmacists are somewhat evenly split among three groups which differ with respect to their attitudes on the three subsets of items. Two of the groups, which constituted 40% of the pharmacists, appear to be fairly neutral toward the general idea of substitution. The most prosubstitution group (agreed with substitution in general, was heavily influenced to substitute, and had little concern about critical dose drugs) consisted of only 13% of the pharmacists.

THERAPEUTIC RECOMMENDATIONS

As previously stated, a therapeutic recommendation occurs when a pharmacist suggests to a patient and/or prescriber that a prescription be changed. Therapeutic recommendations include recommendations for switching to a generic and recommendations for dosing changes, as well as recommendations that a prescription be changed to a therapeutically equivalent but generically inequivalent drug or that a drug not be dispensed at all.

In keeping with the overall goal of drug utilization review, recommendations of this type can be based on economic or clinical factors. Economic factors would include third-party coverage restrictions or price differences between products that are professionally considered to be therapeutically equivalent. The major purpose in making a therapeutic recommendation based on economic factors is to minimize

TABLE 2. Pharmacists' Attitudes Toward Generic Substitution.

	Attitudinal Cluster				
	1 (n = 381) 46%	2 (n = 160) 19%	3 (n = 107) 13%	4 (n = 176) 21%	Total (n = 824)
Generic substitution items	5.7	3.8	6.2	4.7	5.2
a. All products that are rated by the FDA as generic equivalents can be considered therapeutically equivalent with the brand product and each other	5.3	3.0	6.1	4.3	4.7
e. I willingly substitute generics for brand name prescription products	6.2	4.3	6.6	5.1	5.6
j. Few physicians are opposed to the use of generics today	5.7	4.4	5.9	4.7	5.2
k. There is no real difference between most brand products and their generic equivalents	5.7	3.6	6.3	4.7	5.2
Influence to substitute items	6.1	5.8	6.0	4.8	5.7
b. Patients want me to substitute	5.6	4.8	5.8	4.5	5.2
d. Managed care increasingly is forcing pharmacists to dispense generics	6.6	6.6	6.2	5.5	6.3
g. In order to make a profit, I have to dispense generics	5.7	5.6	5.5	3.9	5.3
i. The price difference between generics and brand products is often so great I feel I must offer patients generic substitutes	6.5	6.0	6.6	5.2	6.1
Critical dose drug items	5.1	5.9	2.5	4.5	4.8
c. Therapeutic failures are a serious problem with some generic products	3.9	5.0	1.9	3.6	3.8
f. Dosing on some prescription drugs is too critical to accept the wide range of bioavailability that the FDA allows among generic drugs	5.3	6.1	2.4	4.5	4.9
h. Being required to dispense generics for "critical dose drugs" will increase my exposure to lawsuits	5.0	5.9	2.1	4.0	4.6
l. There are some "critical dose drugs" that I do not think should be substituted even when required by third parties	6.4	6.7	3.5	5.7	5.9

Notes: Letters indicate the order in which the statements were presented in the questionnaire.
   Agreement with statements rated using a 7-point scale where: 1 = strongly disagree and 7 = strongly agree.
Source: Banahan BF III, Kolassa EM, McCaffrey DJ III. Segmentation of retail pharmacists based on attitudes toward generic substitution and narrow therapeutic index drugs. Paper presented at the American Pharmaceutical Association Annual Meeting, 1995.

financial burdens that may affect compliance and to assure the most cost-effective therapy. Through therapeutic recommendations, community pharmacists play an important role in enforcing managed care formularies and performing disease management.

Clinical conditions, such as the detection of a severe drug-drug interaction, are obvious reasons for pharmacists to make therapeutic recommendations. At times, however, pharmacists may be aware of alternative products with more subtle clinical advantages or better safety profiles that, in their judgment, would be "better" therapeutic choices than the prescribed products. In these cases, the pharmacist is assuming the role of a clinical pharmacist in making therapeutic recommendations. Recommendations of this type can be somewhat threatening to the pharmacist-physician relationship, especially when the pharmacist has not previously established a consulting relationship of this type. Because physicians may perceive clinically based therapeutic recommendations as instances of pharmacists questioning physicians' clinical judgment, pharmacists are less confident in making these recommendations.

Pharmacists' Attitudes Toward Therapeutic Recommendations

The differences in pharmacists' attitudes toward therapeutic recommendations based on clinical and cost factors are illustrated by the findings of a 1992 national survey of community pharmacists conducted by the University of Mississippi (Table 3) (9). When asked a series of attitudinal items about therapeutic recommendations, pharmacists more strongly agreed that they should make recommendations for cost reasons than for clinical reasons. In addition, they more strongly agreed that it was appropriate to make recommendations reactively, in response to patients reporting side effects or complaining about costs.

When pharmacists are segmented into attitudinal clusters, approximately half believe that they should make therapeutic recommendations for both cost and clinical reasons, especially when they are doing so in response to a patient complaint about high costs or side effects (Table 3). The remaining pharmacists are fairly evenly split, with 21% agreeing they should make therapeutic recommendations based on cost reasons, but not as much on clinical reasons, and 29% expressing that they did not think it was appropriate to make therapeutic recommendations for either reason.

These results probably depict what is happening with most of the pharmaceutical care issues today. Although a large percentage, perhaps even half, of community pharmacists do believe they should be taking active roles in monitoring and maintaining patients' medication therapy, many pharmacists do not agree with all aspects of the new

TABLE 3. Pharmacists' Attitudes Toward Therapeutic Recommendations.				
	Attitudinal Cluster			
	1 (n = 123) 29%	2 (n = 209) 50%	3 (n = 87) 21%	Total (n = 419)
Patients' advocate a. As a pharmacist, I should serve as patients' advocate for appropriate drug therapy, making reasonable efforts to recommend alternative choices to providers when needed	4.7	6.2	5.5	5.6
Therapeutic recommendations–clinical issues	3.7	5.4	2.8	4.3
n. It is appropriate for me to recommend that a physician change the product prescribed based on perceived clinical advantages of an alternative product	3.3	4.7	1.9	3.7
m. When I believe a patient will have fewer side effects with an alternate medication to the one prescribed, I should contact the physician to discuss the alternatives before I dispense the prescribed medication	3.5	5.5	2.2	4.2
k. If a patient reports problems with side effects and another drug product exists which may be as effective with fewer side effects, I should contact the prescribing physician and recommend the prescription be changed	4.3	5.9	4.2	5.1
Therapeutic recommendations–cost issues	3.4	5.9	5.1	5.0
g. It is appropriate for me to recommend that a physician change the product prescribed based on price differences of alternative products	3.5	5.8	4.5	4.8
c. Even if a patient has not complained about the price of their prescription, if they have a financial hardship and another less expensive but equally effective drug product is available, I should contact the prescribing physician and recommend the prescription be changed	3.2	5.9	5.3	5.0
i. When a patient complains about the price of a prescription and another less expensive but equally effective drug product is available, I should contact the prescribing physician and recommend the prescription be changed	3.6	6.1	5.6	5.3

Notes: Letters indicate the order in which the statements were presented in the questionnaire.
Agreement with statements rated using a 7-point scale where: 1 = strongly disagree and 7 = strongly agree.
Source: Banahan BF III, McCaffrey DJ III. A survey of pharmacists' involvement in medication therapy decisions. University, MS: Research Institute of Pharmaceutical Sciences, 1993.

roles that are being defined for pharmacists. A such, some pharmacists are aggressively implementing these new expanded roles while others are continuing to practice in much the same way they have for the last decade or so. The challenge to pharmaceutical marketers is to identify the innovative pharmacists and to implement strategies for developing effective relationships with these practitioners.

Prevalence of Therapeutic Recommendations

It is difficult to determine the exact frequency with which community pharmacists make therapeutic recommendations because of the nature of the interaction. When a pharmacist determines that a therapeutic recommendation is warranted, he or she contacts the prescriber, explains the situation that is believed to warrant a change in therapy, requests a change in the prescription, and often suggests an alternative product, dosing, etc. If the prescribing physician accepts the recommendation, the pharmacist dispenses the prescription as if it had been written as recommended. When this occurs, the prescribing physician actually has changed the prescription and the new prescription is often recorded as if it had been phoned in by the prescriber. As such, only the new prescription is recorded in the pharmacy management system and in the patient's medication record. Unless the pharmacist plans to submit a claim for reimbursement of the professional intervention performed, the exact number of therapeutic recommendations and the original prescription information usually are not documented.

Although there are no precise estimates of the frequency of therapeutic recommendations made by community pharmacists, several studies have documented the occurrence of the behavior and provide an indication that the behavior is fairly common. In addition to patients becoming actively involved in the selection of generics, they have also become active in ways that encourage pharmacists to make therapeutic recommendations that may lead to switches to alternative products. A 1992 University of Mississippi survey found that 100% of pharmacists report having patients who voice concerns about the price of their prescription medications (17). More importantly, when asked what they did in response to patient complaints about high prescription costs, 56% of the pharmacists indicated they call the prescribing physician to see if a less expensive medication could be prescribed and dispensed; thus they make a therapeutic recommendation that an alternative product be used.

In a 1991 national survey, community pharmacists estimated that they make recommendations that prescriptions be changed to less expensive products five times a week when prescriptions are phoned in and three times a week when they have to initiate contact with the prescribing physician (12). In a subsequent study completed in 1993, 76% of community pharmacists indicated they make therapeutic recommendations to physicians that prescriptions be changed to alternative, equivalent drug products because of the high cost of the medication prescribed (Table 4). This type of therapeutic recommendation based on patient price was estimated to occur 4.4 times per week, with physicians accepting 77% of these recommendations. Pharmacists who report making therapeutic recommendations typically report fairly high rates of physician acceptance.

When these figures are weighted by the prevalence of each type of pharmacy, it is estimated that community pharmacists in the United States make therapeutic recommendations based on cost alone 186,944 times per week. If it is assumed that all of the pharmacists working in these pharmacies make recommendations at this rate and the figures are further weighted by the number of pharmacists working in each type of pharmacy, the number of therapeutic recommendations based on prescription costs is estimated to be 321,697 recommendations per week. Based on the rate of acceptance reported by these pharmacists, the 1993 study estimated that between 143,434 and

TABLE 4. Prevalence of Pharmacists Making Therapeutic Recommendations Based on the Cost of Medications.

	Type of Pharmacy				
	Indep. (n = 212)	Chain (n = 70)	Discount Store (n = 14)	Super-market (n = 26)	Total (n = 322)
Do you ever recommend to a physician that a prescription be changed to an alternative, equivalent, drug product because of the high cost of the medication prescribed?	79%	73%	54%	70%	76%
IF YES:					
Approximately how many times per week does this occur? (mean)	4.5	4.0	4.8	4.4	4.4
Approximately what percentage of the time does the physician accept your recommendation? (mean)	78%	78%	61%	72%	77%
After you make recommendations of this type, do physicians appear to change their future prescribing habits in favor of the less expensive medication? (% responding yes)	48%	39%	50%	38%	45%

Source: Banahan BF III, McCaffrey DJ III. A survey of pharmacists' involvement in medication therapy decisions. University, MS: Research Institute of Pharmaceutical Sciences, 1993.

245,895 prescriptions each week are changed to alternative products due to pharmacists making therapeutic recommendations in response to the high cost of medications. These figures do not include changes made as the result of therapeutic recommendations based purely on clinical issues.

The residual effect of these recommendations on physician prescribing behaviors can be far-reaching. In this 1993 study, 45% of the pharmacists who make therapeutic recommendations based on high prices reported changes in physicians' future prescribing habits in favor of the less expensive medications the pharmacists had recommended. This works much the same way that formulary management works to shape physician prescribing behaviors to conform to the desired formulary.

Therapeutic recommendations made in reaction to patient requests or known clinical problems are the most frequently performed and probably the least threatening to the pharmacist-physician relationship. When a pharmacist makes a therapeutic recommendation in response to a patient behavior or objective therapeutic outcome, the recommendation can be viewed as feedback to the physician. Thus, the pharmacist works as a team member with the physician and the physician-pharmacist relationship is not unduly threatened.

Although reactive therapeutic recommendations are probably the type most frequently made by pharmacists, the number of proactive therapeutic recommendations should increase as pharmacists become more involved in therapy decisions. Proactive recommendations are made without an external stimulus such as formulary restrictions or patient complaints. Disease management is a good example of an emerging pharmaceutical care service where community pharmacists increasingly will be making proactive therapeutic recommendations as they become more involved in evaluating, monitoring, and managing patients' therapies.

Managed Care and Manufacturer Programs
to Encourage Therapeutic Recommendations

Pharmaceutical manufacturers, PBMs, and managed care organizations have all used therapeutic recommendations by pharmacists as a means of influencing drug product selection in efforts to control drug utilization, enforce formularies, or alter market share. Pharmaceutical manufacturer supported programs that have provided reimbursement

to pharmacists for making recommendations resulting in patients being switched to different products have frequently drawn criticism and
have run into problems with the FDA.

Although pharmaceutical manufacturers and PBMs are showing an
increasing willingness to reimburse pharmacists for therapeutic recommendations and other cognitive services, this raises various professional ethical issues. In practicing pharmaceutical care, pharmacists
should be serving as patients' advocates working with patients and
physicians to ensure optimal pharmacotherapy. This involves a clinical judgment and a judgment about what is the most cost-effective
therapy in each situation. Just as recommending a good bioequivalent
generic product can reduce health care costs while maintaining the
same level of therapeutic benefit, recommending an alternative therapeutically equivalent agent can, at times, substantially reduce health
care related costs without negatively affecting therapeutic outcomes.
The potential for conflict occurs when pharmacists are compensated
for successfully switching patients to alternative drug products and
their motives for making the therapeutic recommendation are suspect.

As would be expected, the nature of the recommendation, the form
of reimbursement, and the source of the incentive payment all influence the perceived level of potential conflict of interest. The University of Mississippi examined the issue of professional conflict when
making therapeutic recommendations in a study conducted during
1994 (18). In general, pharmacists reported that receiving higher reimbursement fees for using generics did not present much potential for
conflict of interest, regardless of the source of the reimbursement
(Table 5). However, receiving special reimbursement or higher reimbursement fees for switching patients to alternative products created a
greater potential for conflict of interest. The potential for conflict
varied considerably among the different reimbursement sources, with
Medicaid payments being perceived as having the least potential for
conflict and payments from manufacturers being perceived as having
the greatest potential for conflict.

When the pharmacists in the study were segmented based on their
perceptions of the potential for professional conflict, four groups were
identified. Approximately 30% of community pharmacists were in a
group that perceived very low levels of potential conflict with payments from any source. This group was in stark contrast to the 17% of
pharmacists who reported moderately high or high levels of potential

TABLE 5. Pharmacists' Perceptions of Potential Professional Conflict When Making Therapeutic Recommendations.

	Perceived Conflict Cluster				
	1 (n = 109)	2 (n = 143)	3 (n = 79)	4 (n = 145)	Total (n = 476)
a. You switch a patient from one brand to another lower priced brand product and receive no special reimbursement	1.2	1.6	2.6	1.9	1.8
b. You switch a patient from a brand to the generic of an alternative product and receive no special reimbursement, but you make a greater profit on the alternative product	2.0	2.0	4.3	3.3	2.8
c. You receive a special reimbursement from an HMO/PPO for getting a patient switched to a product on their formulary	3.4	2.4	6.0	5.2	4.1
d. You receive a higher reimbursement fee from an HMO/PPO for dispensing a generic rather than a brand	1.9	2.0	6.0	4.1	3.3
e. You receive a special reimbursement from a PBM for getting a patient switched to a product on their formulary	3.6	2.6	6.2	5.2	4.2
f. You receive a special reimbursement from a PBM for dispensing a generic rather than a brand	2.0	2.2	6.1	4.1	3.4
g. You receive a special reimbursement from Medicaid for getting a patient switched to a product on their formulary	2.2	1.7	6.1	3.8	3.2
h. You receive a higher reimbursement from Medicaid for dispensing a generic rather than a brand	1.6	1.6	5.9	3.1	2.8 ·
i. You receive a special reimbursement from a manufacturer for counseling patients receiving initial prescriptions for their products	2.3	1.4	4.0	2.9	2.5
j. You receive a special reimbursement from a manufacturer for contacting patients regarding lower priced alternatives to medications they are already receiving	5.5	2.2	5.7	4.7	4.3
k. You receive a special reimbursement for detailing physicians about one of the manufacturer's products	5.4	2.5	5.7	4.7	4.4
l. You receive special reimbursement from a manufacturer for successfully getting a patient switched to their products from an alternative therapy	6.0	2.8	6.4	5.4	4.9

Notes: Letters indicate the order in which the statements were presented in the questionnaire.
Potential for conflict rated using a 7-point scale where: 1 = very little potential for conflict and 7 = great potential for conflict.

Source: Banahan BF III, McCaffrey DJ III, Kolassa EM. Community pharmacists' attitudes toward and involvement in therapeutic recommendations and cognitive services reimbursement programs. University, MS: Research Institute of Pharmaceutical Sciences, 1995.

conflict from any special reimbursement for switching patients to generics or alternative products. The other two groups perceived high levels of potential conflict from payments from manufacturers, but differed with respect to whether payments from HMOs/PPOs and PBMs presented a potential conflict of interest. The results of this study reflect the uncertainty that appears to exist among pharmacists and other groups who are struggling to secure reimbursement for cognitive services and pharmacists' interventions while at the same time controlling the potential for conflict of interest in receiving payments for these activities.

Disease Management and the Pharmaceutical Care Movement

A major component of the pharmaceutical care movement is for pharmacists to assume greater roles in monitoring patient therapies and more active roles in assessing treatment outcomes and making interventions and recommendations regarding therapy. One of the direct outcomes of these efforts has been the increased attention given to drug therapy monitoring in general and an increase in pharmacist interventions and therapeutic recommendations.

One of the most exciting areas of the new movement has been the number of pharmacists seeking additional training to prepare for more active clinical roles and for the provision of disease management. A recent national study by the Georgia College of Pharmacy found that over 40% of community pharmacists had participated in one or more postgraduate education programs to develop specialized pharmaceutical care services (19). Smoking cessation programs were the most frequently mentioned (44% of pharmacists), followed by hypertension monitoring (43%), respiratory care (42%), and cholesterol monitoring and screening (34%).

Many independent and chain pharmacies are experimenting with disease management programs. In July 1997, Medicine Shoppe joined forces with CIGNA Health to launch a program that would provide disease management services for peptic ulcer disease and congestive heart failure in 15 Medicine Shoppe pharmacies in the Kansas City area (20). This unique project is designed to collect pharmacy and medical care data that can be used to evaluate the health and economic outcomes of such activities. Although the development of formal disease management programs in community pharmacies is relatively new, early results indicate that these programs can make significant differences in health and economic outcomes. Since providing patient education, monitoring therapy, and making therapeutic recommendations are the crux of these programs, it only stands to reason that pharmacists will become even more influential in product selection and medication use in the future.

IMPLICATIONS FOR PHARMACEUTICAL MANUFACTURERS

The growing role of community pharmacists in prescription product selection presents both opportunities and difficulties for pharmaceutical manufacturers. Difficulties arise in that community pharmacists have historically been viewed by most manufacturers as having little, if any, influence on prescription product selection beyond generic substitution. This view has led many companies to reduce or eliminate calls on community pharmacies by professional sales representatives. As a result, most sales forces are out of touch with what the community pharmacies in their areas are doing with respect to therapeutic recommendations, disease management, and other aspects of pharmaceutical care. Gearing up to call on community pharmacies will not only take additional personnel, but may also require a different message than most sales representatives are trained to deliver today.

The type of product information that will be needed by pharmacists practicing pharmaceutical care–and especially those providing disease management services under contract with patients and/or payers–will present another difficulty for pharmaceutical manufacturers. Disease management services are evaluated based on outcomes and are often reimbursed on a capitated basis. Because of this, pharmacists providing disease management services are more likely to expect pharmacoeconomic and outcomes related data similar to what is needed for pharmacists in managed care organizations. This sales call will be very different from the message and materials delivered to physician practices, thus increasing the difficulty of efficiently managing the sales force.

One of the opportunities these trends present to pharmaceutical manufacturers is that many pharmacists are struggling to determine how and what pharmaceutical care services they are going to provide in their practices. There is a tremendous need for education, training, and assistance with evaluating the outcomes of these new services. This not only provides a mechanism for reestablishing a good relationship with these providers but also provides an opportunity for manufacturers to help shape the way these services are provided in the future. Disease management and focusing on health and economic outcomes is the current trend throughout the health care system. Pharmaceutical manufacturers that can provide the products and services delivering the best outcomes may find that community pharmacists can become strong allies.

REFERENCES

1. U.S. Department of Health and Human Services. Food and Drug Administration. Approved drug products with therapeutic equivalence evaluations. 17th ed. Rockville, MD: DHHS, 1997.

2. Banahan BF III, Tucker PP, Tucker GK, Murphy MN. Trends in hospital pharmacy purchasing and product selection: implications for the drug industry. University, MS: Research Institute of Pharmaceutical Sciences, 1988:4-15.

3. Allnutt RF. PMA's concern about therapeutic substitution. Am Pharm 1990; NS30:39.

4. Grabowski HG, Vernon JM. Substitution laws and innovation in the pharmaceutical industry. Law Contemp Prob 1979;43(1):43-66.

5. Parker RE, Martinez DR, Covington TR. Drug product selection–part 1: History and legal overview. Am Pharm 1991;NS31(7):72-8.

6. Pharmacists are found reluctant to substitute. Am Druggist 1977;121(3):25.

7. Mason JB, Beardon WO. Generic drugs: consumer, pharmacist and physician perceptions of the issues. J Consumer Aff 1980;14(1):193-206.

8. Anon. 1990 national survey of retail pharmacies: summary report. University, MS: Research Institute of Pharmaceutical Sciences, 1990.

9. Banahan BF III, McCaffrey DJ III. A survey of pharmacists' involvement in medication therapy decisions. University, MS: Research Institute of Pharmaceutical Sciences, 1993.

10. Epstein D. Generics: a stronger vote of confidence. Drug Top 1995;(Mar Suppl):6S-12S.

11. Smith MC. Pharmaceutical marketing: strategy and cases. New York: Pharmaceutical Products Press, 1991.

12. Banahan BF III, Jernigan JM. Price sensitivity and generic substitution: a comparison study of physicians and retail pharmacists. University, MS: Research Institute of Pharmaceutical Sciences, 1991.

13. Banahan BF III, Kolassa EM, McCaffrey DJ III. Generic substitution and narrow therapeutic index drugs: a national survey of retail, hospital, managed care, and nursing home pharmacists. University, MS: Research Institute of Pharmaceutical Sciences, 1994.

14. Anon. Consumers still believe in generic drugs, says poll. Med Ad News 1990;9(2):3+.

15. Rankin K. Generics are on the comeback, but can pharmacy trust them? Drug Store News Pharm 1992;2(6):15+.

16. Banahan BF III, Kolassa EM, McCaffrey DJ III. Segmentation of retail pharmacists based on attitudes toward generic substitution and narrow therapeutic index drugs. Unpublished.

17. Banahan BF III, McCaffrey DJ III. Pharmacists' growing influence on MDs' product selection. Pharm Times 1993;59(8):28-40.

18. Banahan BF III, McCaffrey DJ III, Kolassa EM. Community pharmacists' attitudes toward and involvement in therapeutic recommendations and cognitive service reimbursement programs. University, MS: Research Institute of Pharmaceutical Sciences, 1995.

19. Kotzan JA, Martin BC, Poirier S, Nichols G, Perri M, Pritchard L. Pharmaceutical care: community pharmacists' attitudes and practices. Am J Integrated Healthcare 1997;1(1):37-42.

20. Frederick J. Medicine Shoppe stretches boundaries with disease, patient compliance efforts. Drug Store News: Chain Pharm 1997;7(8):1+.

Leveraging Community Pharmacy
to Improve Patient Compliance

David J. McCaffrey III
Noel E. Wilkin

INTRODUCTION

All too often health care providers arrive at a correct diagnosis and devise appropriate management plans, only to be frustrated by unsatisfactory outcomes resulting from the patient not understanding the instructions or in many instances, choosing to ignore them. The efficacy of any treatment depends on the appropriateness of the treatment and the extent to which patients' adhere to the recommended regimen. The consequences of noncompliance with prescribed regimen may be grave, including exacerbation and progression of disability, development of secondary complications, more frequent medication emergencies, unnecessary prescriptions for more potent and potentially more toxic drugs or dosages, and, in general, failure of treatment. If treatment is ineffective, unless adherence to the recommended self-care rec-

David J. McCaffrey III, Ph.D., and Noel E. Wilkin, Ph.D., are Assistant Professors of Pharmacy Administration and Research Assistant Professors in the Research Institute of Pharmaceutical Sciences, School of Pharmacy, University of Mississippi, University, MS 38677.

[Haworth co-indexing entry note]: "Leveraging Community Pharmacy to Improve Patient Compliance." McCaffrey, David J., III, and Noel E. Wilkin. Co-published simultaneously in *Journal of Pharmaceutical Marketing Practice* (Pharmaceutical Products Press, an imprint of The Haworth Press, Inc.) Vol. 1, No. 2 (#2), 1998, pp. 37-60; and: *Marketing to Pharmacists: Understanding Their Role and Influence* (ed: Benjamin F. Banahan III) Pharmaceutical Products Press, an imprint of The Haworth Press, Inc., 1998, pp. 37-60. Single or multiple copies of this article are available for a fee from The Haworth Document Delivery Service [1-800-342-9678, 9:00 a.m. - 5:00 p.m. (EST). E-mail address: getinfo@haworthpressinc. com].

ommendations is measured, it is impossible to determine whether the ineffectiveness was due to the treatment itself or because it was not carried out as instructed. (1)

–Turk and Rudy

If compliance with a therapeutic regimen can have a dramatic impact on the outcomes associated with medication consumption, who stands in the best position to influence these behaviors (or nonbehaviors) and who is the best potential ally for those interested in compliance enhancement? Is it the physician? While the physician is a responsible and influential member of the health care team, because of his or her relative position in the medication-taking process, the physician is at a distinct disadvantage in the war against noncompliance. Is it the patient? While it seems reasonable to direct efforts at the very individuals who are exhibiting noncompliance behaviors, patients' motivation to comply and their ability to read and understand medication information are just two of the many factors that must be considered before such efforts can be undertaken. Is it the community pharmacist? The community pharmacist possesses a unique position with respect to compliance enhancement activities. Why is this the case? First, community pharmacies are accessible to the population: in general, more than 55,000 outlets. Additionally, through the medication patient profile, the community pharmacist has access to detailed medication-taking behavior information that many would consider essential to creating solutions for noncompliant patients. Lastly, pharmacists continue to be considered America's most trusted profession (2). This article concentrates on an area in which the community pharmacist can significantly enhance compliance. This area is prescription-filling behavior.

The ultimate goal of pharmacist intervention is to improve patient drug consumption behavior. Improvement, or appropriate drug consumption, is typically evaluated by comparing drug consumption behavior to the prescribed regimen. The outcome of this evaluation has been called both adherence and compliance. Given that this paper deals with a simple comparison of the behavior to a standard (the drug regimen), it makes no comment on the cause of the behavior. In other words, noncompliance simply means that the observed behavior does not equal the prescribed behavior. This is consistent with the perspective that compliance is the extent to which behavior corresponds with prescribed treatment (3). Inherent in this perspective are the assumptions that (1) a patient must consume a drug to attain optimal health outcomes and (2) the physician is prescribing drugs according to regimens that are proven to be efficacious (or that the pharmacist has intervened to ensure an appropriate drug regimen).

Improvement of drug consumption behavior necessarily begins with identifying the extent to which a mismatch exists between prescribed behavior and actual behavior. Significant work has been conducted to evaluate consumption that differs from the prescribed regimen. The behavior that necessarily precedes consumption is prescription filling.

THE PHARMACIST-PATIENT-COMPLIANCE INTERACTION

Given that noncompliance with drug therapy is defined as the number of doses not taken or taken incorrectly that jeopardizes the expected therapeutic outcome(s), how is it that noncompliant patients present themselves to health care providers (4)? For many, noncompliance behavior is considered an all or none phenomenon. Most frequently, patients are classified as either compliant or noncompliant, and percentages of noncompliant patients are reported and discussed. However, the literature shows that compliance behavior is and should be considered more of a dynamic behavior moving along a continuum rather than a dichotomous behavior.

Fincham and Wertheimer argued that a patient's behavior should never be considered always compliant or always noncompliant (5). They posited a compliance continuum, whereby a patient's behavior may be categorized into one of several types of "compliance" at any given time (Figure 1).

The patient's initial behavior, according to this continuum, is a result of his or her decision to pursue the physician's treatment recommendations (e.g., the prescription). Initial noncompliance is the

FIGURE 1. The Compliance Continuum

Initial noncompliance↔Varying compliance↔Compliance↔Hypercompliance instance whereby patients *do not* receive the medication prescribed for them by physicians. These errors of omission result in an absolute drug holiday and a total loss of the therapeutic benefit that could have been derived from taking the medication. From a marketing perspective, these errors also result in a total loss of sales (failure to realize sales) associated with these prescriptions.

Varying compliance is a result of behaviors that give drug consumption the appearance of being in accordance with the prescribed regimen at times and out of line at others. The designation of compliant is bestowed on patients whose behaviors result in consumption that appears to match the prescribed regimen. The hypercompliance category describes what appears to be overuse of the medication. Patients' prescription-filling patterns can influence all of the categories along the continuum. Filling prescriptions more frequently than prescribed results in a patient being categorized as hypercompliant, for example, while infrequent or sporadic filling behavior is varying compliance. The initial noncompliance category is of particular interest because the patient must possess the drug initially (or initiate therapy) for consumption to take place.

Broadly defined, initial noncompliance is the instance whereby patients, of their own accord, fail to receive the intended medications. Initial noncompliance should be thought of as two distinct phenomena–unpresented prescriptions and unclaimed prescriptions.

Unpresented prescriptions are those prescriptions issued by the physician but neither delivered to the pharmacy (pharmacist) by the patient or the patient's agent nor delivered to the pharmacy through the physician's office (e.g., phoned-in, facsimile, electronic transfer, or mail). An *unclaimed* prescription is any prescription that has been presented in a pharmacy (either by the patient or an agent of the patient or phoned-in to a pharmacy), whether filled by the pharmacist or not, for which the patient does not wait or return to pick up, arrange to have picked up, or have delivered.

Once a patient has received a prescription and begun therapy, health care professionals are generally interested in measuring the varying degrees of compliance with the therapy. Usually this is done by measuring noncompliance. On a micro level, noncompliance is measured as the number of doses taken correctly (i.e., at the correct time, in the correct amounts). More frequently, noncompliance is measured on a macro level through an analysis of refill behavior over time with the metric being an estimate of the number of days without therapy divided by the number of days the patient was considered to be on therapy.

Although this classification of the different types of noncompliance helps in organizing a review of the topic, the distinctions between the different types of compliance are often not as clear as these definitions would imply. For this reason, it helps to view behavior for individual patients as a more dynamic process, with compliance being a result of patient behavior at different points throughout a patient's course of therapy with a specific agent. As illustrated in the following discussion of the different compliance categories, behaviors that result in initial noncompliance affect compliance after therapy has been initiated. The following sections of this paper are intended to provide a somewhat detailed review and discussion of some of the more important reasons why a compliant or noncompliant result was obtained when patient behavior was compared to the prescribed regimen. It also identifies areas in which pharmacists have the greatest potential to improve patient behavior that results in enhanced patient compliance.

Unpresented Prescriptions

Unpresented prescriptions technically include both new prescriptions of which the pharmacist has no knowledge and authorized refills that are not requested. Unpresented *new* prescriptions are most often what people refer to with the term unpresented prescriptions and can be thought of as those prescriptions that are typically pocketed by patients. The unpresented *refill* prescription is related to the varying compliance outcome and will be discussed in a later section.

The earliest published work on unpresented new prescriptions was performed in the early 1960's by Hammel, Campbell, and Williams at the University of Wisconsin. The authors found that 2.4% of all prescriptions issued in a Midwestern town of 3,000 remained unpresented 10 days after issue (6). Additionally, the researchers found that 83% of the unpresented prescriptions were written, whereas only 17% were phoned-in to the pharmacy. The researchers followed up on all unpresented prescriptions to uncover why the patients were noncompliant. The patients stated that they did not need the medication at the time the prescription was issued but planned to have it filled later, they had some of the same medication at home, or they did not feel a need for the medication. The authors also concluded that the price of the prescription had no effect on the likelihood of a patient filling a prescription.

Hammel and Williams continued work in the area in 1964 by conducting a four-phase study auditing prescription files of pharmacies located within communities of differing populations at different times of the year to offset any potential seasonal effects (7). They found the overall incidence of unpresented prescriptions to be 3.3% 10 days after issue. They also noted unpresented rates ranging from 0.5% to 4.9% for the different populations but found no association between population size and incidence of unpresented prescriptions. The researchers followed up on the noncompliant patients to determine the reasons for initial noncompliance. Thirty-four percent of initially noncompliant patients reported that they had no need for the medication, while 11% reported having medication at home. Also noteworthy is that 45% of the initially noncompliant patients had their prescriptions filled more than 10 days following issuance. Finally, the authors reported that anti-infectives, sedatives, dermatologicals, and analgesics made up approximately 50% of all unpresented prescriptions. As in the authors' previous work, cost was *not* mentioned as a reason for patients failing to fill their prescriptions initially.

Taubman and colleagues reported the overall incidence of unpresented prescriptions to be 6% in an urban clinic in Detroit, Michigan (8). They went on to suggest that a possible method of minimizing initial noncompliance would be use of a quadruplicate prescription form. The distribution of the form would be as follows: one copy would remain in the physician's office, one copy would be sent to billing, one copy would go to the pharmacy (i.e., prescription), and the fourth copy would be collected to allow intervention in those cases where initial noncompliance was suspected.

Waters, Gould, and Lunn investigated unpresented prescriptions in a mining practice in Hatfield, Great Britain. Using the National Health Service prescription forms (FP10), the investigators found an overall rate of unpresented prescriptions of 7% (9). Additionally, they found the lowest rate (3%) among elderly nonpaying patients and the highest rate (26%) among paying men aged 25-34 years. Furthermore, they found that the noncompliance rate decreased in patients exempt from the 20p per item charge. This study was the first to show any evidence of a possible association between price and rate of unpresented prescriptions.

Luckman and colleagues discovered the rate of unpresented prescriptions to be 6% for patients suffering from upper respiratory infection, urinary tract infection, hypertension, or diabetes (10). They discovered that the rate of what they called Level 1 noncompliance increased with treatment of acute disease states. They also found a relationship between ease of access to pharmacy (convenience) and a higher compliance level. Further, they found that frequent patient contact for a specific disease tends to increase initial compliance.

Rashid found the rate of unpresented prescriptions 30 days after issue to be 20% in Preston, Great Britain (11). The author also found that psychotropics and anti-infectives were the most frequently represented drug classes among the unpresented prescriptions and that the rate of unpresented prescriptions increased in lower socioeconomic classes. Interestingly, Rashid reported that 65% of all prescriptions written were filled within 48 hours.

Begg found that 6.4% of a month's prescriptions issued in a semiurban area of Scotland remained uncashed (unpresented) 6 months after issuance (12). Additionally, he discovered that those patients required to pay for their prescriptions (i.e., possessed no exemption) were almost three times as likely not to have their prescriptions filled.

Krough and Wallner found that 10 days after issue, 7% of prescriptions remained unpresented in a metropolitan clinic in Minneapolis, Minnesota (13). Colored prescription blanks were used to track prescriptions. All pharmacies within the study area were asked to provide data about those prescriptions filled. Noncompliant patients were contacted by phone to determine if the prescription issued to them was, in fact, filled. In addition to the 7% confirmed unpresented prescriptions, 15% of the prescriptions written could not be tracked; thus, the rate of initial noncompliance might be significantly greater.

During 1985, The Upjohn Company commissioned a national survey investigating compliance. As a part of this study, 1,020 consumers were contacted and asked questions regarding their compliance behaviors. Fourteen percent of the respondents reported that they had received a prescription within the last 12 months yet chose not to have it filled (14). The most cited reasons for not having a prescription filled were: did not need it (51%), did not want to take it (21.7%), and cost (10%). Comparison of noncompliance rates across family income also provided interesting results. People in the middle income range ($15,000-$24,999) reported the highest rate of initial noncompliance.

This might be expected due to the fact that the lower income and low middle income families are more likely to be receiving public assistance, thus reducing, if not eliminating, the cost of prescriptions. The survey found no association between gender and age groups and the reported incidence of unpresented prescriptions. This same type of investigation was conducted in 1988. The percentage of respondents indicating that they had received a prescription and elected not to have it filled rose to 20% (15). Younger customers (less than 60 years of age) were more likely to report not having a prescription filled. When asked why they did not fill the prescription, more than one-half of the respondents reported that they did not need the medication. One-third of those believing that they did not need the medication stated that the reason for this decision was that they felt better.

Saunders reported that 20% of patients discharged from the emergency department failed to fill their prescriptions within 24 hours (16). No differences in compliance were found based on gender or method of payment. The reasons for noncompliance were reported to have been cost, lack of transportation (i.e., convenience), and negligence. The product classes most frequently unpresented were antibiotics and analgesics. It should be noted, however, that the definition of initial noncompliance for this study was any prescription not filled within 24 hours of receipt. The incidence of noncompliance would be likely to decrease if an alternative criterion–perhaps 5 to 10 days–was used.

Schering Laboratories produces an ongoing series of research studies designed to explore the major issues affecting the profession of pharmacy. Schering Report IX examined several improper compliance issues. The report showed that 7% of patients who received a prescription following a physician visit did not have it filled (17). The survey found that compliance increases with an increase in the number of prescriptions taken. Only 5% of the elderly (over age 40) were found to be initially noncompliant; this increases to 10% in patients under 30. Also surprising was the finding that college graduates were reported to have a higher rate of initial noncompliance (6%) than those without high school diplomas.

In 1992, Schering Laboratories repeated (but not in its entirety) the 1987 study. This report revealed that 8.7% of patients who received a prescription following a physician visit failed to have that prescription filled (18). In comparison with the results of the previous study, the 1992 study showed a 1.7% increase in initial noncompliance as reported by consumers. The 1992 report failed, however, to show any difference in the reasons patients fail to fill their prescriptions.

Pequet found that 20% of the elderly had failed to fill a prescription (19). This rate is quite high. What might be more alarming is that the study showed that the physician is mostly ignorant of the initial non-compliance behavior.

In another investigation of uncashed prescriptions in Great Britain, Beardon and colleagues tracked 20,921 issued prescriptions and found that 14.5% of those patients receiving prescriptions failed to redeem them at a pharmacy (20). These 14.5% of patients accounted for just over 5% of all issued prescriptions (1.5 prescription items per patient). A higher percentage of patients without exemption (i.e., free prescriptions) failed to have their prescriptions filled, as did female patients. Higher percentages of initial noncompliance were found for prescriptions written on Friday, Saturday, and/or Sunday.

Galloway and Eby conducted a national survey of impoverished residents to investigate potential nontraditional roles for the pharmacist. They asked the respondents, "For those times you failed to have a prescription filled, why?" The reasons given were as follows: cost (financial reason), did not need it, and felt better (21). Those 3 reasons made up almost 70% of all responses for initial noncompliance in the impoverished.

These findings indicate that patients are making assessments as to the value or benefit of having a prescription filled (and possibly as to whether they should consume the medication), i.e., they seem to be assessing the need for the medication. This assessment is likely to take the cognitive form of a belief or perception. While studies have found relationships between initial noncompliance and factors other than need, such as age, disease state, cost, education, and the day of the week, it is possible that these correlations are being driven by patients' beliefs regarding the need for a medication (9, 10, 12, 15, 17, 20). The lower rate of initial noncompliance in the elderly could be due to their trust in their physician, which may lead them to believe that if the doctor wrote the prescription then they need it. It is reasonable to assume that the sicker one is, the more intense the belief that a medication is needed. This is consistent with finding a lower initial noncompliance rate in acute disease states (10). Regarding cost, it can be postulated that a patient must really believe that he or she needs a medication to pay a high price for it, which would account for the relationship between initial noncompliance rate and cost. More well-educated people might be more likely to feel comfortable assessing their need for a medication, resulting in a higher rate of initial noncompliance in college graduates, as found in Schering Report IX (17). The association between the day of the week and need is more tenuous. However, it is plausible that after waiting until Monday to fill the prescription written on Friday, Saturday, and/or Sunday, the patient no longer believes the medication is needed. These assertions are just that–assertions–and need to be subjected to empirical study. The results can have significant implications for how patients are educated when they receive an order for a prescription.

From the standpoint of initial compliance enhancement, there is very little, if anything, that community pharmacists can do to address the unpresented prescription phenomenon. It is unrealistic to think that pharmacists can intervene when they are unaware of the problem. However, as the use of electronic transmission of prescriptions from the prescriber to the pharmacy increases, unpresented prescriptions can be eliminated completely. Overall, compliance rates may not increase because electronic submission of the prescription would only move the prescriptions from a classification of unpresented to one of being unclaimed, but making the pharmacist aware of the prescription at least improves the chances for intervention. Potential intervention activities directed toward unclaimed prescriptions are discussed in the following section.

Unclaimed Prescriptions

An unclaimed prescription is any prescription which has been presented in a pharmacy, either by the patient or an agent of the patient, or phoned-in to a pharmacy, whether filled by the pharmacist or not, and for which the patient does not wait or return to pick up, arrange to have picked up for him or her, or have delivered. The studies addressing initial noncompliance are concentrated in the unpresented new prescription area. Although unpresented prescriptions do have an impact on the pharmacy's net profit, the unclaimed prescription has additional effects of lost pharmacist time, lost opportunity costs, and potentially higher inventory costs.

The first known work done in the area of unclaimed prescriptions was performed by Katz and Segal at the University of Toronto. By auditing a year's worth of prescriptions not retrieved from the outpatient pharmacy of a large Toronto general hospital, the authors found that approximately 0.5% of all prescriptions went unclaimed (22). This number is quite low given the percentages found in the literature, possibly because the survey was conducted in Canada, which has a national health service. The lack of expenditures prior to having a prescription filled might, in fact, increase the number of prescriptions retrieved from the pharmacy. The authors also found that anti-infectives (21.3%) and central nervous system agents (18.1%) made up the largest percentage of unclaimed prescriptions. Fifty-five percent of unclaimed prescriptions were prescribed for females and 45% for males. Additionally, the number of unclaimed prescriptions decreased as the distance traveled to reach health care outlets increased.

Fincham and Wertheimer have investigated initial noncompliance in the elderly population. In 1986, they found an unclaimed prescription rate of 0.28% for elderly patients enrolled in a large Midwestern health maintenance organization (HMO) (23). In 1988, the authors attempted to elicit the reasons the elderly failed to claim their medications. By surveying those elderly who had unclaimed prescriptions in the pharmacy of a large Midwestern HMO, they found that acute disease states and convenience items (cost, proximity to pharmacy, long wait, special trip, and possession of a supply of the medication) were most frequently mentioned (23). For those patients burdened with chronic disease, the feeling that the drug was not needed was the most often mentioned reason for not claiming medications.

Craghead and Wartski conducted a study to investigate the effect that an integrated hospital computer system would have on the number of unclaimed prescriptions. The baseline rate of unclaimed prescriptions was reported to be 1.5% (24). Following implementation of the computer system, they found that the rate of unclaimed prescriptions increased to 1.85%. Additionally, they found the rate of unpresented prescriptions declined approximately the same percentage. The implementation of an integrated computer system had no net effect on initial noncompliance. Although the system successfully reduced the number of unpresented prescriptions, it increased the number of unclaimed prescriptions, thus placing an additional burden on the pharmacy department. In 1991, the authors published a study that concentrated on which drug classes appeared frequently as unclaimed prescriptions. The rates of unclaimed prescriptions within general drug categories per total unclaimed prescriptions were: anti-inflammatories (17.5%), prenatal care products (13.0%), antibiotics (9.2%), and cough and cold preparations (5.2%) (25).

Farmer and Gumbhir, auditing the prescription files of 21 pharmacies in and around Kansas City, Missouri, found that the mean age for *all* prescriptions was 45.62 days (26). The majority of these unclaimed prescriptions (81%) were telephoned into the pharmacy. Additionally, anti-infective agents (17%), cough and cold preparations (11%), topicals (9%), analgesics (8%), and nonsteroidal anti-inflammatory agents (7%) made up over half of all unclaimed prescriptions. The authors also reported that only 26% (5 of 21 pharmacies) credited third parties for unclaimed prescriptions.

Ring, in a master's thesis written at the University of Cincinnati, found the rate of unclaimed prescriptions to be 0.63% in a convenience sample of 59 metropolitan Cincinnati retail pharmacies (27). In a calculation of the cost associated with each unclaimed prescription, the investigator found that a $5.67 loss occurred. Therefore, unclaimed prescriptions not only caused losses due to the unrealized sale but also incurred almost $6 per unclaimed prescription in pharmacist time and materials. Additionally, the author found that pharmacists did not view the unclaimed prescription phenomenon as a problem and that pharmacists believed it would be difficult to reduce the number of prescriptions that go unclaimed.

McCaffrey investigated the rate of unclaimed prescriptions on a national sample of retail pharmacies (28). Overall, pharmacists reported the rate of unclaimed prescriptions to be 0.87%. Chain pharmacies (12.60) experienced a rate of unclaimed prescriptions nearly double that of independent pharmacies (6.60). The results also showed that private-pay customers were perceived to contribute most to unclaimed prescriptions. This result added legitimacy to the pharmacists' belief that cost is a contributing factor in the unclaimed prescription phenomenon.

Kirking and Kirking investigated the rate and composition of unclaimed prescriptions at the University of Michigan Ambulatory Care Pharmacy. Overall, they found that 1.2% of all prescriptions remained unclaimed 7 to 13 days following receipt by the pharmacy (29). Additionally, they found that topicals, central nervous system products, and anti-infectives were the most represented drug classifications among the ranks of the unclaimed. Interestingly, 64% of all unclaimed prescriptions were picked up within 30 days, leaving a final rate of unclaimed prescriptions after 30 days of only 0.5%.

In a continuation of their 1993 investigation, Kirking and Kirking, along with Zaleon, found 522 unclaimed prescriptions (1.6%) for 344 patients in an ambulatory care pharmacy (30). Of those 522 prescriptions, 185 were claimed by patients within 21 days and 337 (1%) were unclaimed after 3 weeks. The elderly (65+) had the highest rate of unclaimed prescriptions (81.8%). In all instances, prescriptions written for discharge patients were more likely to be found in the ranks of the unclaimed.

Most recently, a national unclaimed prescription audit was undertaken to deepen understanding of the unclaimed prescription phenomenon (31). The study tracked 15,478 prescriptions filled or received by the investigation pharmacies as to their disposition over a 30-day period. Of these prescriptions, 96.2% were claimed within 48 hours of receipt by a pharmacy. The remaining 589 were tracked, and all but 191 were claimed within 30 days (a rate of 1.5%). Independent pharmacies experienced a much lower rate of unclaimed prescriptions than chain pharmacies (1.04 and 1.80, respectively). Somewhat surprisingly, patients continued to claim prescriptions up to 26 days after the pharmacy's receipt of the prescriptions.

The underlying behaviors that account for the results obtained regarding unclaimed prescriptions are not easily distilled. The evidence suggests that the belief in the need for a medication still plays an integral role (5). In addition, the finding that anti-infectives predominate this category provides some evidence that need is playing a role. It is plausible that patients believed that they had a need for the medication when they presented it, but that belief changed before the medication was picked up. However, findings that contradict the role of need, [e.g., the finding that the elderly have a greater rate of unclaimed prescriptions (30)] make it more difficult to assert that it accounts for the largest amount of variance in these findings. It is likely that systematic variables can also account for a portion of these results (e.g., ability to present the prescription, but inability to get it picked up). Unfortunately, these findings do not provide much guidance in the way of intervention development. Further empirical research on this phenomenon is necessary to develop efficient and effective interventions into unclaimed prescriptions, an area of great interest to pharmacists and the pharmaceutical industry. Pharmacists have the potential to affect unclaimed prescriptions, as they possess the information necessary to influence this phenomenon, have the ability to develop the patient relationship necessary to influence patient behavior, and have enough contact with the patient to implement effective interventions to alter unclaimed prescription rates.

Unpresented Refill Prescriptions

Unlike unpresented new prescriptions, unpresented refills are similar to unclaimed prescriptions in that pharmacists are aware of them and do have the opportunity to affect patient refilling behavior. Several studies have investigated the refill rates in community pharmacies. Hammel found that in a chronically ill population, refill compliance decreased each month. At the end of 6 months, only 44% of prescriptions for antihypertensive medications were dispensed.

Schering Report IX found that 32% of those surveyed reported that they had not refilled a prescription that their physician had ordered (17). Additionally, 50% of the patients recalled being given instructions by the physician to have their prescription refilled. Only 20% recalled a pharmacist giving such information (18).

Schultz and Gagnon investigated 100 randomly selected pharmacies to assess the degree to which available refills were obtained by patients (32). Tracking 1,058 prescriptions (no 0 refill or PRN medications) from each pharmacy, they found that roughly half (54%) of the authorized refills were ever dispensed.

Baird, Broekmeier, and Anderson investigated the effectiveness of a computer-assisted refill reminder system on refill compliance rate (33). They found that the refill reminders did have a significant effect (improvement) on the rate of compliance with refill prescriptions (18.6%). Despite this impressive gain, the most important information from the investigation was that 86% of refill prescriptions for cardiovascular agents and 82% of refill prescriptions for all medications available for refill were not dispensed.

Simkins and Wenzloff assessed the effectiveness of postcard and telephone refill reminder systems. They found that the refill reminders were effective in reducing the rate of refill noncompliance; however, like Baird and colleagues, the authors failed to realize the significance of the overall percentage of patients not complying with physicians' instructions to refill medication (> 40%).

Fedder tracked the disposition of 120,000 prescriptions in 5 suburban Baltimore, Maryland, pharmacies. He found that 77% of authorized refills were never activated (34).

Skaer and colleagues, analyzing 1 year's prescriptions for 128 patients covered under the South Carolina Medicaid program, found that refill reminders and special packaging significantly improved compliance (35). Over the course of 1 year's time, patients received 232.5 days of therapy. Translated into refill compliance terms, 35% of refills were not dispensed.

In the research described above, the number of unpresented refills ranges from 35% to 86% of authorized refills. This tremendous number raises several questions. Why aren't patients refilling the prescriptions in instances where the physician has authorized refills? Do the patients believe that these medications are not needed? Were the patients simply prescribed another medication that supplants their need for the medication with authorized refills (are these statistics a false alarm)? These are empirical questions that need to be explored. Pharmacists need to have a better understanding of what these high rates of unpresented prescriptions signify. Assuming that these are useful indicators of patient filling behaviors (and ultimately of drug consumption behavior), the findings regarding unpresented and unclaimed prescriptions can have significant implications for the health of the patients, the profitability of the pharmacy, and the profitability of the pharmaceutical industry.

IMPLICATIONS OF UNCLAIMED AND UNPRESENTED PRESCRIPTIONS

The implications for unclaimed and unpresented prescriptions can be categorized according to the impact that these phenomena have on the patient, the pharmacy, and the pharmaceutical manufacturers.

Impact on the Patient

The considerable amount of unpresented and unclaimed prescriptions is one indicator that patients may be experiencing suboptimal drug therapy. Of course, this is based on the assumption that if the patient had received and consumed the unpresented or unclaimed prescription, it would result in more optimal drug therapy. If a patient never fills a prescription that would result in improved health status, obviously an optimal drug therapy outcome has not been achieved and suboptimal drug therapy results. The true impact of these phenomena on health outcomes needs to be evaluated empirically. In any case, these phenomena can be used by the pharmacist as indicators of patient behavior. More importantly, their existence provides an opportunity for the pharmacist to discuss the patient's drug consumption patterns and behavior. More research in this area is necessary to understand the significance of unpresented and unclaimed prescriptions with regard to health outcomes and how pharmacists can use these indicators most effectively in their efforts to achieve optimal drug therapy with every patient.

Impact on Pharmacy

While it is understood that the health and well-being of the patient is of the greatest concern for the pharmacist, the financial aspects of noncompliance need to be investigated by pharmacists as well, especially those owning their own practices. Just as suboptimal drug consumption has a negative impact on patient outcomes, it can have an adverse effect on the fiscal health of community pharmacies. However, through efforts designed to improve compliance with recommended treatments, pharmacists can significantly improve the financial health of their pharmacy while improving patients' chances of arriving at optimal therapeutic outcomes. Table 1 shows the potential impact that capturing unpresented refills would have on the gross

TABLE 1. Increase in Net Profit from Increased Refill Compliance.*					
% Increase in New Refills	Number of Renewals	Revenue Increase	Gross Margin**	Variable Expense*	Increase in Net Profit
5%	18,583	$20,036	$5,830	$2,605	$3,225
10%	19,468	$40,072	$11,661	$5,209	$6,452
20%	21,238	$80,145	$23,322	$10,418	$12,904
30%	23,007	$120,195	$34,977	$15,625	$19,352
40%	24,777	$160,268	$46,638	$20,835	$25,803
50%	26,547	$200,341	$58,299	$26,044	$32,255

* Adapted from: Jackson RA, Huffman DC. Patient compliance: the financial impact on your practice. NARD Journal 1990;112(Jul):67–71.
** Based on 29.1% of sales
*** Estimated to be 13% of sales

profit of a hypothetical pharmacy and, for some, the added impetus it would provide for incorporating a refill reminder program into their pharmacy practice.

Research reveals that between 5% and 10% of all written prescriptions are never presented to a pharmacy for filling. This figure, combined with the estimated 2 billion prescriptions written in the United States alone, will result in the "loss" of between 100 million and 200 million prescriptions annually. Using a conservative estimate of the average prescription price [$26.48], the revenue that is not realized by community pharmacy lies between $2.6 billion and $5.2 billion annually (36).

Because of the manner in which initial noncompliance is manifested, pharmacists are not aware of the specific behaviors that lead to noncompliant outcomes in the case of unpresented new prescriptions. As a result, the pharmacist is almost powerless to take action to correct this undesirable health behavior. The pharmacist has the opportunity, through global messages as to the importance of pharmacotherapy, to influence a patient's attitude toward having new prescriptions filled. However, the responsibility of recognizing and changing initially noncompliant behaviors, as it relates to unpresented new prescriptions, must lie with all interested parties (i.e., the physician, the pharmacist, the pharmaceutical manufacturer).

Unpresented prescriptions are not only new prescriptions that have been issued by physicians but also all refill prescriptions remaining in the patient profile that have not been activated by the patient or the pharmacist. While they have no control over unpresented new prescriptions, pharmacists do have the opportunity to affect compliance with refill prescriptions. Once the pharmacy receives a prescription or a prescription has been identified as needing to be filled, the pharmacist can and must become a major force in correcting initially noncompliant behavior.

Like the unpresented prescription, the unclaimed prescription has the potential for deleterious effects on pharmacy revenue (Table 2); however, it has associated with it unique characteristics that make it worth considerable pharmacy attention. First, the unclaimed prescription differs in the evidence the pharmacist has that an aberrant health behavior has taken place. Typically, the pharmacist has evidence that aberrant health behavior has taken place from the fact that the filled prescription remains in the pharmacy.

TABLE 2. Economic Impact of Unclaimed Prescriptions (Adjusted for Pharmacy Type and Prescription Volume).

Pharmacy Type	Per Pharmacy Daily Rx Volume	Per Pharmacy Annual Rx Volume	Unclaimed Rx Rate	Per Pharmacy Annual Unclaimed Rx
Independent	112	34,942	1.04	363
Drugstore Chain	179	62,775	2.16	1,356
Discount-Rx Dept.	155	53,570	1.36	728
Grocery-Rx Dept.	130	45,526	1.55	705

Pharmacy Type	Number of Outlets (U.S. Total)	Number of Unclaimed Rx by Type	Estimated Retail Worth ($26.48/prescription*)
Independent	24,862	9,024,906	$238,979,510
Drugstore Chain	17,270	23,418,120	$620,111,817
Discount-Rx Dept.	4,837	3,521,336	$93,244,977
Grocery-Rx Dept.	6,274	4,423,170	$117,125,541
Totals	53,243	40,387,532	$1,069,461,845

* – 1994 NARD-Lilly Digest Average

An additional characteristic makes the unclaimed prescription an important issue for community pharmacy. In the majority of cases, these prescriptions are prepared for dispensing and are waiting for the patient to claim or arrange for delivery. Considering the time expended in the preparation of many of these prescriptions, the costs associated with the unclaimed prescription, at least for the community pharmacy outweigh the costs of the prescription that was never presented.

As for the future, more than 90% of pharmacists indicated that they thought the number of unclaimed prescriptions had remained unchanged (76.2%) or had increased (14.9%) (31). Without successful intervention, the unclaimed prescription will continue to have a dramatic financial impact on community pharmacy.

Impact on the Pharmaceutical Manufacturers

The impact of unpresented and unclaimed prescriptions on the pharmaceutical manufacturers is primarily economic. It is manifested in three ways: lost revenue, inappropriate use, and physician beliefs. When patients do not present or claim prescriptions that have been ordered, the results are fewer units of medications sold. This has a direct financial impact on the pharmaceutical manufacturer in the form of lost revenue. The influence of these drug consumption behaviors could be underestimated if we only consider the losses at face value. Although no research exists as to the likelihood of filling subsequent prescriptions after a noncompliance episode, in all likelihood, subsequent authorized refills will also be lost. Additionally, future sales of the product can be influenced by inappropriate filling and consumption behavior. When a physician prescribes a medication for a patient, he or she assumes that the patient had the prescription filled and consumed the medication as prescribed. If the patient does not fill (and consume) the medication as prescribed and his or her condition worsens, then the physician may assume that the drug was ineffective. The physician's belief about the effectiveness of the medication and future prescribing of the drug are likely to be affected. As a result, one unpresented or unclaimed prescription could have a far greater impact on product sales and company profitability than originally suspected. An additional concern is the risk that other prescribers will be influenced by the attitudes of this one physician. Diffusion from one physician to other physicians has the potential to elevate the influence of an unpresented or unclaimed prescription on the revenue of the pharmaceutical industry. Ultimately, drug consumption behavior, including filling behavior of the patient, is the primary factor that moderates the correlation between drug efficacy and drug effectiveness. This fact warrants the further study of unclaimed and unpresented prescriptions for the purpose of developing means to ensure drug effectiveness.

The pharmacist is the health care professional who has access to the data necessary to evaluate unpresented and unclaimed prescriptions, has sufficient contact with the patient to influence prescription filling patterns, and has the respect sufficient to influence patient behavior. Pharmacists are therefore logical partners for the pharmaceutical industry and physicians in the effort to improve patient filling and drug consumption behavior. For pharmacists to be effective, research is needed to develop an understanding of the true meaning of these indicators and to develop interventions that are proven to affect patient filling behavior. Education to improve pharmacists' use of prescription data is also necessary.

MEASUREMENT OF SUBOPTIMAL
DRUG CONSUMPTION

A means of measuring and a solid understanding of indicators such as unpresented and unclaimed prescriptions would be of great value to pharmacists. The profession still lacks a viable means of evaluating unpresented new prescriptions. Technology that links the physician to the pharmacist will be necessary to capture the full magnitude of this phenomenon and to develop interventions to improve patient presenting behavior. Once a prescription is on file in the pharmacy prescription management system, the pharmacist has the data necessary to generate indicators that drug consumption does not correspond to the prescribed regimen. One such strategy available to the community pharmacist is the refill reminder.

Refill reminder systems can automatically contact patients due to have their prescriptions refilled through the use of a computerized phone system. Other systems provide reports that generate postcards to patients, and still others give the pharmacist the information necessary to contact the patient personally. There is some evidence that refill reminder systems have the ability to enhance the correspondence between what was prescribed and patients' filling patterns [e.g., (37)]. However, it is not understood how these systems are altering filling behaviors. There are many questions that remain about this technology and the cause of its impact on patient filling behavior. These questions include, "Which refill reminder system has the greatest impact on patient behavior, computerized or personal systems?" "How does the refill reminder system influence patient behavior, is it through influencing the belief that the medication is needed and/or important?" "Is the influence of these systems moderated by the level of credibility or trust that is bestowed on the pharmacist by the patient?" Further, well-designed studies are necessary to provide pharmacists with guidance on this issue. Until the true impact is known, monitoring patient refill behavior still serves a valuable purpose for the pharmacist. Through monitoring, the pharmacist has an opportunity to approach the patient about his or her drug therapy. This provides an opportunity to explore drug consumption patterns, experiences with the medication, and current health status. As pharmacists become more involved in patient care, these opportunities will become more valuable.

Despite the evidence that supports recapturing these prescriptions as a revenue and profit generating enterprise and their usefulness as a clinical tool, a study performed in the early 1990's found that only 6% of computerized pharmacies and 5% of manual pharmacies sent refill reminders to their patients (38). More recently, results from a national community pharmacy survey found that 14.3% of all community pharmacies (18.3% of chain pharmacies and 11.1% of independent pharmacies) are using some form of refill reminder system (39). QS/1 Data Systems and Condor Corporation were two of the first pharmacy computer systems companies to introduce refill reminder programs as a service to users. According to a *ComputerTalk* survey, one-third of chains reported having similar refill reminder programs operating in their stores (40).

The basic technique used in most of these programs is that the prescription database is used to identify patients who are late getting a refill (noncompliant), and a reminder letter or phone call is used to notify the patient. In most of the systems, if the prescription has still not been refilled after a period of one or two weeks, a second letter or phone call is used to notify the patient somewhat more firmly. If this reminder fails, the patient is labeled as a chronic noncomplier and is dropped from the refill reminder program.

Unfortunately, these tools are only as good as the data collected. Evidence suggests that pharmacists need to evaluate the quality of the data before relying on the contents of the database to identify and contact patients regarding their drug consumption behavior. Banahan and Bentley found the percentage of incorrect days' supply information, for example, ranged from 0% to 36.9% in their sample (41). These indicators will only be as good as the data that comprises them.

In recent years, pharmaceutical manufacturers have shown an increased interest in compliance. Much of this interest has been focused on how compliance enhancement can be used to increase sales. Manufacturers' compliance enhancement programs primarily provide information, rebates, and coupons to the patient through the mail. It is not yet clear how these programs have an effect on patient drug consumption behavior. This is not to minimize the role of the pharmaceutical industry in this arena. The sales of its products, the health of patients, and appropriate use of its products are at stake. Through a better understanding of these readily accessible indices, the pharmaceutical industry could facilitate the development of targeted and effective interventions to affect unpresented and unclaimed prescriptions.

CONCLUSION

Deviations in drug therapy from the regimens found to be efficacious in clinical trials have and will continue to make health professionals strive to improve drug consumption behavior. Many tools and indicators assist health professionals to identify those patients who seem to be consuming medications in a manner that differs from what is prescribed. Unclaimed prescriptions and unpresented prescriptions are such indicators. However, like other indicators of patient behavior, further understanding of these phenomena would help in the development of pointed and effective interventions to improve the specific behaviors that lead to suboptimal drug consumption in the general population. Until then, pharmacists must proceed by individually addressing the needs of each patient and determining what is necessary to optimize the patient's drug therapy.

REFERENCES

1. Turk DC, Rudy TE. Neglected topics in the treatment of chronic pain patients–relapse, noncompliance, and adherence enhancement. Pain 1991;44(1):5-28.

2. Still number one. NARD J 1997;119(2):22-3.

3. Haynes RB, Taylor DW, Sackett DL, eds. Compliance in health care. Baltimore: Johns Hopkins University Press, 1979.

4. Smith DL. Patient compliance: an educational mandate. Norwich, NY, and McLean, VA: Norwich Eaton Pharmaceuticals, Inc., and Consumer Health Information Corporation, 1987.

5. Fincham JE, Wertheimer AI. Elderly patient initial noncompliance: the drugs and reasons. J Geriatr Drug Ther 1988;2(4):53-62.

6. Hammel RW, Campbell NA, Williams PO. Unfilled prescriptions in your pharmacy? J Am Pharm Assoc 1961;NS1(3):155-7.

7. Hammel RW, Williams PO. Do patients receive prescribed medication? J Am Pharm Assoc 1964;NS4(7):331-7.

8. Taubman AH, King JT, Weisbuch JB, Little F, French D. Noncompliance–in initial prescription filling. Apothecary 1975;9(10):14-46.

9. Waters WHR, Gould NV, Lunn JE. Undispensed prescriptions in a general mining practice. Br Med J 1976;278:1062-3.

10. Luckman R, Weisbuch JB, Taubman AH, King J, Little F, French DM. Drug compliance–a study of patient behavior based on medical records. Drug Intell Clin Pharm 1979;13(Mar):136-43.

11. Rashid A. Do patients cash prescriptions. Br Med J 1982;284:24-6.

12. Begg D. Do patients cash prescriptions? An audit in one practice. J R Coll Gen Pract 1984;34:272-4.

13. Krough C, Wallner L. Prescription-filling patterns of patients in a family practice. J Fam Pract 1987;24:301-2.

14. Primary reasons why prescriptions are left unfilled by pharmacy customers. Kalamazoo, MI: The Upjohn Company, 1987.

15. National pharmacy service study. Kalamazoo, MI: The Upjohn Company, 1988.

16. Saunders C. Patient compliance in filling prescriptions after discharge from the emergency department. Am J Emergency Med 1987;5(4):283-6.

17. The forgetful patient: the high cost of improper patient compliance. Schering Report IX. Kenilworth, NJ: Schering Laboratories, 1987.

18. Improving patient compliance: is there a pharmacist in the house? Schering Report XIV. Kenilworth, NJ: Schering Corporation, 1992.

19. Pequet BK. Prescription drugs: a survey of consumer use, attitudes, and behavior. Washington, DC: AARP, 1984.

20. Beardon PHG, McGilchrist MM, McKendrick AD, McDevitt DG, MacDonald TM. Primary noncompliance with prescribed medication in primary care. Br Med J 1993;307:846-8.

21. Galloway SP, Eby CE. Poverty area residents look at pharmacy services. Am J Public Health 1971;61:2211-22.

22. Katz EF, Segal HJ. Unclaimed prescriptions. Hosp Admin Can 1971;(Nov): 50-4.

23. Fincham JE, Wertheimer AI. Initial drug noncompliance in the elderly. J Geriatr Drug Ther 1986;1(1):19-29.

24. Craghead RM, Wartski DM. Effect of automated prescription transmittal on number of unclaimed prescriptions. Am J Hosp Pharm 1989;46:310-2.

25. Craghead RM, Wartski DM. An evaluative study of unclaimed prescriptions. Hosp Pharm 1991;26:616-32.

26. Farmer KC, Gumbhir AK. Unclaimed prescriptions: an overlooked opportunity. Am Pharm 1992;NS32(10):55-9.

27. Ring PE. The unclaimed prescription phenomenon as an additional pharmacy operation burden [Thesis]. Cincinnati, OH: University of Cincinnati, 1991.

28. McCaffrey DJ III, Smith MC, Banahan BF III, Juergens JP, Szeinbach SL. The financial implications of initial noncompliance: an investigation of unclaimed prescriptions in community pharmacies. J Res Pharm Econ 1995;6(1):39-64.

29. Kirking MH, Kirking DM. Evaluation of unclaimed prescriptions in an ambulatory care pharmacy. Hosp Pharm 1993;28:90-102.

30. Kirking MH, Zaleon CR, Kirking DM. Unclaimed prescriptions at a university hospital's ambulatory care pharmacy. Am J Health-System Pharm 1995;52:490-5.

31. McCaffrey DJ III. Initial noncompliance: the definition and description of the unclaimed prescription phenomenon in community pharmacy. A national unclaimed prescription audit pilot [Dissertation]. University, MS: University of Mississippi, 1995.

32. Schulz RM, Gagnon JP. Patient behavior patterns regarding prescription refills. Unpublished.

33. Baird TK, Broekmeier RL, Anderson MW. Effectiveness of a computer supported refill reminder system. Am J Hosp Pharm 1984;41:2395-7.

34. Fedder DO. The pharmacist and cardiovascular risk reduction. U.S. Pharm Cardiovasc Dis Suppl 1990;(June):4-8.

35. Skaer TL, Sclar DA, Markowski DJ, Won JKH. Effect of value-added utilities in promoting prescription refill compliance among patients with hypertension. Curr Ther Res 1993;53:251-5.

36. 1994 NARD-Lilly Digest. Indianapolis, IN: Eli Lilly and Company, 1994.

37. Simkins CV, Wenzloff NJ. Evaluation of a computerized reminder system in the enhancement of patient medication refill compliance. Drug Intell Clin Pharm 1986;20:799-802.

38. Banahan BF III. What are you doing with that computer? ComputerTalk 1993; 13(1):6-8.

39. Pulse of Pharmacy™. The 1996 National Survey of Community Pharmacy Management and Operational Practices. University, MS: University of Mississippi, 1996.

40. Pumping up your profit flow. ComputerTalk 1996;16(4):15-23.

41. Banahan BF III, Bentley JP. Information management practices that support pharmaceutical care service. Drug Top 1996;(Sept 16):98-107.

Pharmacists and Disease Management

Robert E. Martin

INTRODUCTION

Historically, the pharmaceutical industry has focused on physicians as the primary directors and providers of patient care. Pharmaceutical marketing and research efforts continue to channel the stream of changing technology through physicians as the chosen target group to enhance effective clinical practice and to institute the new equilibriums that occur after new product introduction. Recently instituted care management programs have shown that the physician community can actually pose a barrier to developing care management programs and to implementing current innovations due to the physician's overwhelming workload, outside influences of multiple managed care organizations, PBMs, formularies, and administrative responsibilities.

In developing marketing strategies, pharmaceutical manufacturers have often overlooked the pharmacist. Because of their unique proximity and accessibility to the patient, pharmacists are positioned as valuable players in the design and delivery of what are now becoming known as "care management programs" in the outpatient setting. Although by definition care management programs involve planning and implementation by numerous participants, including inpatient and

Robert E. Martin, M.S., is a consultant with Stuart Disease Management Services.

Address correspondence to: Robert E. Martin, 2377 Gold Meadow Way, Suite 100, Gold River, CA 95670.

[Haworth co-indexing entry note]: "Pharmacists and Disease Management." Martin, Robert E. Co-published simultaneously in *Journal of Pharmaceutical Marketing Practice* (Pharmaceutical Products Press, an imprint of The Haworth Press, Inc.) Vol. 1, No. 2 (#2), 1998, pp. 61-80; and: *Marketing to Pharmacists: Understanding Their Role and Influence* (ed: Benjamin F. Banahan III) Pharmaceutical Products Press, an imprint of The Haworth Press, Inc., 1998, pp. 61-80. Single or multiple copies of this article are available for a fee from The Haworth Document Delivery Service [1-800-342-9678, 9:00 a.m. - 5:00 p.m. (EST). E-mail address: getinfo@haworthpressinc.com].

outpatient clinicians, pharmacists can play an important role on the care management team by providing a unique outpatient pharmacotherapeutic perspective that emphasizes patient advocacy as its primary goal.

This goal of this article is to encourage the utilization of pharmacists to proactively spearhead or participate in the development and negotiation of care management contracts and programs, to function as critical coordinators and monitors of the outpatient care segment of these programs, and to offer their skill and knowledge as the pharmacotherapeutic experts on the care management team. Because care management is a term broadly (and often indiscriminately) used by various health care entities, this paper will begin with this author's definition of care management. It will then explore in more detail the specific process and tasks of care management, how to analyze and select therapeutic areas for development of a care management program, and how the type of care management agreement will determine the pharmacist's involvement in specific interventions. The paper will then describe how disease-specific interventions are developed and implemented. Finally, a case example applying all of these ideas specifically to the pharmacist will be presented. This discussion includes important factors to consider when financial remuneration is expected for pharmacist services rendered as part of a care management team, as well as potential synergistic partnerships with clinical practitioners, key third-party payers, and product and service vendors. The overall goal of this paper is to assist the pharmaceutical industry in identifying ways to utilize the pharmacist in the dynamic evolution of health care delivery. First, however, we must ensure as the foundation of our discussion a common level of understanding by beginning with a detailed definition of care management.

DEFINITION OF CARE MANAGEMENT

As stated previously, care management has been defined in many ways and is misunderstood by many health care organizations (1). True care management requires broad application of disease-specific interventions and behavioral strategies across all health care environments (systemwide) that are designed to improve the efficiency of health care delivery, targeting both providers and the patient. The goal of these interventions is to maximize the end result of patient health (clinical outcomes) while minimizing the cost of delivery of health care (decreasing inappropriate resource utilization). This is achieved by prospective development of a contract specifying who is responsible for what and includes a detailed outline of processes that focus on clinical effectiveness, system efficiencies, resource utilization, and quality of life outcome targets. Again, true care management includes analysis, development, and implementation of interventions across all possible delivery environments involved in a disease state (system-wide) and is not limited to individual components or episodes of care.

Of course the environment (such as an outpatient ambulatory care clinic, inpatient hospital setting, community pharmacy practice, or physician provider group) defines the specific components or interventions of care management that might be undertaken by a particular provider or institution. However, an individual community pharmacy, hospital, or physician provider group acting on its own does not fully represent the care of an individual patient. The patient actually is treated within the unity of the entire health care system. Therefore, in defining the scope of care management, it is necessary to consider the entire health care system of delivery, not just an individual component of care distribution. By definition, care management occurs within a mutually agreed upon, specific time frame, with agreed upon cost and outcomes targets, through the modification or enhancement of provider and patient behavioral interventions.

THE PROCESS OF CARE MANAGEMENT

Because drugs offer themselves as one of our most cost-effective tools in preventing disease, treating disease, and maintaining good health, one cornerstone of care management is pharmacotherapy and the application of pharmacoeconomics. Pharmacoeconomics may be defined as "the description and analysis of the costs of drug therapy to healthcare systems and society" (2). Historically, pharmacoeconomic research has been of limited value to care management because it has focused almost exclusively on double-blind, placebo-controlled, clinical trial type comparator studies of Drug A vs. Drug B. The results of these highly artificial analyses have not lent themselves to the practical application of pharmacoeconomic principles in a real-world population. As we have already stated, true care management needs to be approached from a total systemwide health care perspective rather than from a limited and artificial double-blind, placebo-controlled, clinical trial perspective. Broad opportunity exists for pharmacists to work with managed care organizations, various provider groups such as IPAs and physician practice management groups, and the pharmaceutical industry to perform real-world pharmacoeconomic analyses as a critical component of successful care management programs. All of these groups are demanding real-world pharmacoeconomic analyses to promote utilization of the most effective pharmaceutical products, to justify increasing pharmaceutical costs, and to identify the appropriate place of pharmaceuticals in effective patient care.

Many principles and specific steps of pharmacoeconomics are applicable to the care management process on a broader scale. The key to any successful care management program is measurement–measurement of how a system of providers is currently treating a specific disease state (in terms of resources utilized, clinical parameters, and costs) and measurement of how those patterns of treatment, overall patient health, and costs change once a care management program has been implemented. It necessarily follows that to measure we must be able to retrieve medical and pharmacy encounter data from health system databases. Unfortunately, medical databases in particular are highly limited in their ability to offer useful information regarding clinical parameters, accurate diagnosis and procedure codes, and true costs. As currently available technology is increasingly applied to the creation of clinical data repositories, computerized patient medical records, and real-time accessibility to systemwide, integrated databases for all participants of health care delivery, our ability to design and implement truly effective and sophisticated care management programs will be greatly enhanced. Database studies will increasingly allow us to develop plan-specific and patient-customized health care economic models of disease-specific areas that focus on clinical effectiveness, improved treatment practice guidelines, standardization of patient care, decreased morbidity and mortality, and greater cost control from more efficient resource utilization with emphasis on wellness and prevention.

A critical component of care management is the ability to monitor outcomes. The final assessment of program effectiveness should not only be measured in terms of impact on resource utilization and cost but also in terms of clinical health status and quality of life outcomes of the targeted population. This implies the need for a benchmark database to compare historical treatment of patients with post-intervention treatment of patients. Post-intervention patient outcomes will be compared to historical patient outcomes (the benchmark) to provide assessment of the value and impact of the care management program on resource utilization, clinical effectiveness, and quality of life.

The care management process involves three stages. The first stage is development of a therapy intervention framework (3). The second stage is formal development of a care management agreement. The third stage focuses on implementation and monitoring of that agreement.

In Stage One, the objective is to use existing data from the health care system to analyze practice and treatment patterns, resource utilization, and cost profiles and to use these data to identify cost drivers and patient groups who would be the target of an intervention strategy. In Stage Two, the process of contract negotiation involves profiling resource utilization and costs, formalizing intervention and behavior modification strategies, and agreeing on performance targets (e.g., a capitation rate in a risk-bearing disease intervention) as the basis for estimating program effects on resource utilization and cost structures. Finally, Stage Three focuses on the implementation of the agreement by ensuring that adjunct data collection protocols are followed, that any formulary changes are accommodated within the agreement structure, that targets are evaluated and tracked, and that there are no surprises at the end of the contract period (e.g., agreeing on the cost savings that are to be shared) (4). We will now look more closely at the specific tasks involved in progressing through each of these three stages.

TASKS INVOLVED IN CARE MANAGEMENT

Task I. Development of a Therapy Intervention Framework for the Disease Intervention

The purpose of this task is to establish a therapy intervention modeling framework to identify–for the database made available–the principal treatment pathways, the process of treatment in each pathway (who is responsible for what, when, and how it is performed), the resources used to support treatment, and the associated cost profiles for the treatment population. Such a model not only drives data assembly but also identifies possible care management intervention points, the resource saving and efficiency options, and the appropriate outcomes of therapy. This framework should be linked to established national treatment or other guidelines and to the proposed intervention strategy.

Task II. Establishment of Disease Parameters for Modeling the Disease or Therapy Interventions

This task involves translating Task I into an operational form so that the impact of the proposed intervention can be evaluated in simulated quantitative terms–both in resource units and costs–where medical and pharmacy dimensions are identified. Key cost drivers should be identified (e.g., emergency room visits, drug combinations) and the model used to point to the potential cost savings from behavioral change by both patients and providers.

Task III. Assessment of Database Accessibility and Content

As stated previously, health system databases historically have been notoriously lacking in the capture of clinical parameters, accurate diagnoses, and procedural coding information. These databases also have not been fully integrated in a real-time format that is readily accessible to all health care providers. It is essential for the care management team to evaluate the location, accuracy, and retrievability of needed resource and cost data elements, not just for the preliminary benchmarking analysis, but also for ongoing care management program monitoring and measurement.

Task IV. Issues of Data Collection and Storage

The team must explore and develop practical, efficient tools to locate and collect needed resource and cost data elements in a timely, repeatable manner. Otherwise, the care management program may collapse into a one-time, massive endeavor to collect benchmark data, irreproducible on a consistent, ongoing basis. Consistently reproducible, ongoing data collection and analysis is necessary for continuous monitoring of program impact on resource utilization and costs. Ideally, data collection methods should utilize on-line technology as much as possible to minimize reliance on laborious, manual paper processing (which could also likely deter provider participation and compliance with the care management program). Additionally, the team must also consider the issue of data storage, particularly as it relates to patient confidentiality. Issues for consideration should include amount of data to be collected, the storage medium, confidentiality, and retrieval by all involved practitioners, security, and maintenance (5).

Task V. Database Evaluation and Impact Assessment

Once data from relevant databases is in hand, estimating program impact on resource utilization and cost profiles can be used to test the operational form of the model developed under Task II. Part of this involves database screening to identify relevant resource items, to link these items to diagnostic categories, and to develop an audit trail so that any impact analysis and claims for cost savings can be validated.

Task VI. Development of Resource Utilization Profiles

The term "resource utilization" encompasses all health care resources used to support prevention and treatment of all aspects of a specific disease state. It is important to agree upon resource utilization profiles as a baseline for any disease intervention strategy. Underpinning the modeling in Task V is the identification of resource utilization profiles by treatment pathway and patient characteristics (e.g., age, sex, comorbidities). Agreement on these is essential for any contract negotiation.

Task VII. Development of Cost Profiles

The next step is to translate the outcome of Task VI into cost terms. The purpose is to assess the extent to which costs vary among patients and providers and establish the basis for such cost variation. Cost drivers and the source of cost variation should be assessed via economic modeling because it is important to identify the independent or marginal contribution of particular treatment events (e.g., emergency room visits) to variations in the overall cost of care.

Task VIII. Preparation of a Preliminary Submission

A very important step in the development of a care management program is the submission of a plan to the party who will be reimbursing the program for its efforts. The key in any submission is to make the case for the impact of a particular intervention strategy, given the patterns of resource utilization and costs identified in Tasks I through VII. This means that the analysis must be system-specific, must be transparent, and must provide sufficient detail regarding the assumptions underlying any claim for cost savings and the outcomes for the treatment population.

Task IX. Initiation of the Care Management Agreement

The individual or team who has spearheaded development of a care management program to this point is now ready to begin negotiations with one or more potential partners to establish a care management agreement. The form of the agreement is not fixed. It may be a risk-sharing or risk-bearing (capitated) agreement covering all resources used to support therapy or only a subset of medical and/or drug resources to support a particular intervention. The negotiating parties must reach agreement on the previous tasks undertaken in preparation of the preliminary submission, as well as on the resource utilization profiles, cost profiles, and choice of outcome targets. During the actual negotiation of a care management agreement, Tasks X through IV must be accomplished.

Task X. Agreeing on the Intervention Area or Patient Group

Central to any care management intervention package is agreement upon the target patient group or intervention area and the process by which these patients will be identified. These may be a subset of those initially analyzed for the preliminary submission (e.g., high-risk or high-cost patients), or there may be intervention strategies tailored to different patient groups within a disease area.

Task XI. Agreeing on Target Patient Characteristics and Risk Factors

The intent of Task XI is to repeat Tasks VI and VII for the specific target patient groups to be addressed in the agreement. This step is basically a refinement of what was accomplished in Tasks VI and VII, such that a resource utilization and cost profile can be agreed upon–

specific to the target population–and the resource or utilization elements that are to be the target of the agreed upon strategy can be identified.

Task XII. Agreeing on Outcome Parameters

Using the outcome parameters identified for a specific disease area under Tasks I and II, the team then selects those outcome measures that can be operationalized, the measuring instrument, targets for measured outcomes, and how these data are to be assembled. These outcome measures can include clinical targets, health status targets, and quality of life targets–with agreement reached on the measuring instrument. Outcome parameters will also include resource and cost savings targets, but these should not be developed in isolation.

Task XIII. Agreeing on Intervention Strategies

Given that a case has been made in the preliminary submission for the anticipated quantitative impact of particular (and proprietary) strategies on patient outcomes (with supporting data), the actual intervention strategy is agreed upon, together with materials such as treatment guidelines for physicians and patient education packages, as well as the role and composition of care intervention teams.

Task XIV. Contract Design and Agreement

At this point, the care management team and the payer are ready to draw up a contract. The contract should include:

1. The type of contractual agreement being agreed to
2. A statement of the specific care management objectives
3. Identification of the target patient group for the care management intervention
4. The time frame for retrospective analyses to establish contract cost baselines
5. Profiling of the disease or therapy areas and agreement on data definitions
6. Requirements for resource costing and the identification of cost drivers

7. Seasonal adjustment procedures
8. Agreement on outcome measures, instruments that will be used to measure outcomes, and data assembly techniques
9. Agreement on performance targets
10. Agreement on management and arbitration or dispute resolution procedures. (6)

The last point is worth emphasizing because of the complexities that accompany the performance measures in care management agreements. Unless the agreement is managed appropriately and the parties have agreed to an arbitration process (ideally, compulsory arbitration through a third party), there is a risk of extended litigation in the resolution of disputes. A care management agreement is not static. New drugs are entering the formulary, new techniques are being introduced, and the characteristics of the treatment population may also change as a result of mergers and contracts for new patient groups. A process whereby these elements are accommodated must be part of the natural evolution of the agreement over a specified contract period. Once an agreement concerning the contract period, time lines for interventions, and target outcomes is in place, the implementation phase has to be managed. This involves three tasks: initiation, management, and evaluation of the agreement against contract targets.

Task XV. Initiating the Agreement

Assuming that all materials have been agreed upon and guidelines developed, both parties need to agree on a timeline for introducing the program, given the resources that have been agreed upon to support the intervention. These are essentially process requirements, but it is important that the timeline is followed because performance will depend on it. Quality control is important at this juncture, and a log of provider and patient contacts needs to be kept. Where outcomes are being assessed via a patient longitudinal or panel sample, this needs to be established on an agreed-upon timeline.

Task XVI. Managing the Agreement

A cohesive management group must be assembled. This governing body must agree upon procedures and the basis on which arbitration of disputes will occur (if not stipulated in the contract).

Task XVII. Monitoring the Outcomes

The contract will have specified the outcome targets and measuring instruments. It is important to ensure that data inputs are being received in a timely manner, are in the appropriate format, and are integrated with the medical and drug claim data (4). The ability to adequately monitor and assess the outcome of the interventions is directly related to the accurate and timely application of the required measuring instruments and the collection of medical and cost information.

SELECTING THERAPEUTIC AREAS FOR POSSIBLE CARE MANAGEMENT PROGRAM DEVELOPMENT

Medical and pharmacy claims databases are the main source of information for any retrospective assessment of treatment patterns, identification of the principal cost drivers in treatment, and the profiling of high-risk and potentially high-risk, high-resource utilization patient groups (7). Pharmacy claims data provide an excellent resource for developing a list of targeted therapeutic categories to focus intervention strategies and outcomes monitoring. Any therapeutic area commanding large dollar volumes of resource expenditures is a potential target for care management program development. Also, P&T Committee feedback, patient surveys, practitioner surveys, logs of patient and/or practitioner complaints, and other database analysis (such as hospitalization and emergency room admission rates) can be used to identify potential disease states for care management program development.

Pharmacy claims processors routinely generate reports for health care plans that identify top therapeutic areas by (1) total dollars spent on prescriptions per month and (2) volume of prescription claims per month within specific therapeutic areas. Various systems, such as the American Hospital Formulary System (AHFS), are used in claims processors' on-line systems to classify drugs into specific therapeutic categories, such as cardiovascular, anti-infectives, peptic acid disease, antidepressants, antihyperlipidemics, etc. Once total dollars spent and total volume of prescription claims have been identified for a specific therapeutic category, numerous reports are also provided that drill down to more detailed levels of analysis. These more specific reports can include, but are not limited to, dollars spent and total volume for specific drugs (by brand or generics, strength, and dosage form), top patient utilizers of these drugs, top physician prescribers of these drugs, etc. These reports provide valuable drug product utilization information that can be used as surrogates to identify top cost and resource utilization areas for further analysis by the care management team to identify potential areas where efficiency of care, resource utilization, and resulting costs could be enhanced by implementation of a care management program.

Using pharmacy claims to identify potential areas for care management program development has its limitations. Pharmacy claims serve as surrogate markers only and tell little about an individual patient's health status. In some disease states, high utilization of appropriate pharmaceutical products is desirable, such as in asthma and diabetes. In other disease states, high pharmaceutical use can indicate inappropriate diagnosis and treatment, such as with oral antidepressants or broad-spectrum antibiotics. Pharmacy claims analysis should be used wisely as a guide for further exploration into other health care databases that may reveal more clearly the actual state of appropriate or inappropriate health care delivery.

SELECTING DISEASE-SPECIFIC INTERVENTIONS

There are three types of contractual arrangements that may define the scope of pharmacist involvement in care management. Type I agreements are "full-cost" agreements; that is, the parties agree to either capitate or risk share on the total of all medical and drug costs associated with a disease state or therapy intervention. Type II is a hybrid form under which a portion of the medical costs and all drug costs are covered. Under this agreement, the parties might select only the principal cost drivers in a disease intervention (e.g., emergency department visits or hospitalizations or pharmacotherapy) and contract to reduce them in unit as well as in dollar terms. Finally, Type III is a drugs-only agreement, the purpose of which is to reduce formulary costs–typically through drug switching or by imposing guidelines for drug utilization.

Type III is the least preferred of the types because it offers no guarantee of more efficient allocation of health care resources or of total cost reductions in the health care system. However, Type III agreements may be the most amenable form of care management for implementation by a pharmacist, as the pharmacist is likely unable financially to assume risk for comprehensive medical and pharmacy costs of large groups of patients.

For Type III agreements, patients can be selected via pharmacy encounter claims data. The most appropriate way of identifying patients would be through collection and analysis of integrated medical and pharmacy encounter claims databases (6). However, due to the difficulty of pharmacists accessing the medical encounter databases, a surrogate analysis could be developed through the use of claims data in specific pharmacotherapeutic categories. Appropriate interventions or therapeutic switching programs can be developed for specific patients identified from specific therapeutic areas.

Asthma can be used as an example. In asthma, the lack of medical encounter claims would not preclude us from identifying patients for intervention strategies. Searching NDC codes of antiasthma drugs and other pharmacotherapeutic indications utilized in treating asthma could identify patients. Resource utilization associated with other comorbidities could be eliminated from the data by recognizing pharmacotherapeutic indications that are commonly used in these comorbid conditions (i.e., COPD). These surrogate databases would then allow identification of patients for educational, sociobehavioral, and diagnostic-therapeutic treatment interventions. These patients could also be categorized for appropriate intervention strategies by severity indexing them according to drug utilization. As an example, asthma patients who could be categorized in a high severity index could be those receiving beta agonists, orally inhaled steroids, oral corticosteroids, and leukotriene inhibitors in combination therapy. Patients more appropriately placed at the low end of a severity scale might have a drug profile of beta agonist medications only.

To repeat, however: community pharmacists should be cautious when using pharmacy claims as a surrogate marker for individual patient health status. Severity indexing by resource utilization may not necessarily correlate accurately with the patient's health status, and this would have to be investigated further upon patient enrollment into an intervention program.

One important final consideration in performing data analysis to identify patient populations for intervention programs is the time frame of data analyzed. At least 24 months of data are needed to identify with certainty patients who routinely utilize observable patterns of health care resources (e.g., pharmacotherapy only, pharmacotherapy plus occasional ER visits, hospital admissions). Analyzing data over a short period may miss some patients who should be targeted for intervention, such as patients with clinically severe disease who are not compliant with therapy or patients who have been previously diagnosed but are currently stable (8).

THE INTERVENTION PROCESS

Once patients have been identified and categorized according to severity indices, specific intervention strategies tailored to patient needs can be developed. Health risk assessment (HRA) tools, particularly disease-specific HRAs providing self-reported information, can reveal useful information about the patient's understanding of his or her disease state, skill and knowledge of the treatment process, and ability to self-manage. These tools can be used in combination with claims data analysis to build a disease-specific model that can predict which patients may eventually utilize high-cost resources (e.g., an emergency room visit or hospital admission). The goal is to try to prospectively target these patients *before* they fall into patterns of inefficient health care resource use. These patients can then be targeted for intervention with an intensive program customized to their specific needs to prevent such events.

One of the most effective ways to manage moderate to severe categorized patients is by utilization of a disease-specific intervention team composed of practitioners who are assigned specific roles in the delivery of the patient's care, depending on their specialty (primary care physician, physician specialist, clinical pharmacist, nurse educator, nutritionist, etc.). As stated previously, the pharmacist's unique proximity and accessibility to the patient on a continuing basis may pinpoint the pharmacist as the most appropriate leader of this team in the outpatient setting.

Specific examples of interventions include, but are not limited to, patient education materials and classes, newsletters, videos, disease-specific "tool kits," disease-specific diaries for patients to record symptoms and drug use, pharmacy compliance programs, physician compliance programs, home health care, and specially structured physician visits that include customized surveys, disease-specific treatment guidelines, and further educational materials. The goal is to focus on the patient as the primary manager of his or her own disease state and provide him or her with practical, user-friendly tools that will help with effective self-management. The pharmacist can play a critical role each time the patient returns to the pharmacy for a drug refill by reinforcing appropriate medication use and technique (e.g., inhalers for asthma or injections for migraine) and by reviewing the patient's home management plan. Some managed care organizations are beginning to train and credential select pharmacists as disease-specific educators for diseases like asthma, diabetes, and hypertension. Specific patients are then referred to these pharmacists for individualized care.

CASE STUDY

To discuss more specifically the pharmacist's role in care management, we will now examine a case study to illustrate the principles and issues previously described. The first task of a pharmacist desiring to develop or participate in an effective care management program is to establish potential contractual relationships with a group or groups of capitated providers or capitated third-party payers (i.e., pharmacy benefits managers) who are motivated to improve effective delivery of patient care and contain costs. A substantial amount of preliminary discussion, exploration, and assessment may need to take place before the specific role and responsibilities of the pharmacist within such a group of providers or payers can be established, including financial remuneration for his or her services. The pharmacist who establishes a working relationship with key third-party payers–particularly in securing a formal role as a credentialed provider of specific health care services on a team consisting of other plan providers–is far more likely to be financially reimbursed. Given the scope and depth of work required in effective development, implementation, and ongoing monitoring of a disease management program, the pharmacist would do well to research opportunities for formal contractual relationships to ensure financial remuneration for his or her work.

Either as part of the preliminary analyses, or as part of a formal role within the group, the pharmacist can first assist these providers in performing a retrospective analysis of surrogate pharmacy claims data utilizing NDC codes of disease-specific medications to identify potential therapeutic areas for program development, as well as to generate lists of specific patients of the capitated provider group for intervention. For purposes of this case study, we will assume that the pharmacist and partnering provider group have identified asthma as a disease state where enhancements in care delivery could result in substantial, relatively immediate returns, both clinically and financially. The pharmacist could then assist in segmenting patients into severity index categories based on extended patterns of resource utilization interventions (specifically, by examining the utilization profiles of pharmacotherapeutic agents, i.e., beta agonists only for mild severity indexed patients; beta agonists, orally inhaled steroids, and oral steroids for the highest severity-indexed patient). The next step could be for the pharmacist to coordinate analysis of the provider group's principal treatment pathways of asthma treatment to assess appropriateness of therapy. The pharmacist could also administer asthma health risk assessment surveys directly to the patient population. Results could be stratified to categorize patients into a matrix based on severity of illness and self-management skills.

If the provider group's treatment pattern of this population is determined to be inappropriate, the pharmacist is now provided with the opportunity to coordinate a panel of select community providers, i.e., allergy and/or asthma specialists, pulmonologists, respiratory therapists, nurse educators, to develop a set of clinical practice guidelines to assist in standardizing delivery of appropriate patient care. The purpose of developing and implementing written clinical practice guidelines is to decrease practice variability, potentially related treatment failures, associated inefficient resource utilization, and unmanaged costs.

The guidelines that are developed should be based on national guidelines that reflect the standard of practice not only in the community but also across the country. Starting with a nationally recognized template will greatly reduce the time that would be required if guidelines were developed without a baseline and will lend clinical credibility and acceptance within the local provider community. The pharmacist can assist in this process by locating and distributing copies of nationally recognized guidelines to panel members and coordinating meetings to review and modify these guidelines to meet local practice standards and needs. Once the panel has completed a preliminary draft of the disease-specific guidelines, this draft should be disseminated to specialists and local medical groups for feedback regarding content and applicability to their patient populations. A time limit should be established for this review, and the pharmacist can be instrumental in facilitating all phases of review, including draft distribution and collection of feedback. Once the guidelines have been accepted within the local medical community, the pharmacist can continue the role of facilitator by coordinating the printing and distribution of the guidelines and monitoring ongoing compliance with them.

Effective implementation of an asthma disease management program depends on accurate assessment of individual patient level of knowledge about his or her disease process, self-management, health status, resource utilization, and home environment, as well as the presence or absence of a care management plan. If no care management plan exists between treating physician and patient, the pharmacist has another opportunity to provide patient education and case management and work with community clinicians, home health care agencies, and possibly pharmaceutical industry representatives or employer groups to develop a care management plan and other types of intervention strategies.

Additionally, it would be helpful to establish training and credentialing programs for selected pharmacists in the community to play the role of asthma educator or case manager. Specific patients could then be referred to these pharmacists for individualized asthma care programs by provider groups, employer groups, or managed care organizations. Extending care to the ambulatory care setting within the pharmacy environment could take place within the community pharmacy or within a large medical group practice with an ambulatory clinic focus. This setting would enable the pharmacist to provide care in a specialty care environment with the capacity to provide these services to large numbers of asthma patients.

OTHER TYPES OF INTERVENTION STRATEGIES

Patient Education

Ideally, all patients with asthma, regardless of severity categorization, would receive individualized asthma education. Educational materials, in both written and video form, should be provided to both patients and caregivers. The materials presented by the pharmacist should place emphasis on proper medication use, home monitoring, and establishment of home management plans for asthma exacerbations.

Pharmacy Compliance Program

Pharmacists can play an integral role on the health care delivery team because of their knowledge of pharmacotherapies and their accessibility to patients. Through this program, each time a patient fills a prescription, pharmacists can reinforce medication use, demonstrate proper inhaler technique, and review asthma home management plans with the patient.

Home Health Care

Patients with a high severity index who have previously been regarded as treatment failures due to noncompliance with their asthma care resulting in increased resource utilization would be candidates for referral to this service. An asthma management team in this environment could consist of a respiratory therapist, a pharmacist, and possibly a nurse educator, with the following responsibilities:

1. Monitoring for environmental triggers
2. Providing home respiratory therapy
3. Counseling on medication use
4. Monitoring of pharmacotherapy and care management intervention compliance.

Asthma Classes

Patients with severe asthma could also be targeted for additional education in the form of asthma classes or a dedicated asthma program with a variety of intervention-case management programs, including a pharmacy compliance program (telemonitoring), asthma classes, newsletters, videos, asthma kits, environmental surveys, and focused care management plans during clinic or provider visits. Patients with concomitant asthma and allergies should receive the same interventions intended for patients with severe asthma. Additionally, when possible, the pharmacist could work with employer groups to create asthma group care management programs that are supported at the employees' work site. These programs involve self-care management training offered by respiratory therapists and/or community pharmacists and include self-monitoring of pulmonary function by correct use of peak flow meters.

SUMMARY

The pharmaceutical industry needs to recognize that pharmacists can and do participate in the dynamic evolution of health care delivery by becoming familiar with and applying care management program principles. Traditionally, pharmacoeconomics has been used to analyze the cost impact of drug therapy on the health care system and society but has been limited in its perspective to the randomized clinical trial with comparator analysis of Drug A vs. Drug B. This limited focus has historically reduced its applicability to actual clinical experience in a real-world patient population. Care management programs provide an opportunity for the pharmaceutical industry to expand cost-analysis studies to a real-world setting by systematically gathering the required health resource utilization and outcome information while performing a specified intervention.

The three stages of the care management process described previously (identifying, intervening, and monitoring) may be used by the pharmacist as a structure to guide development of the tasks and activities required for a successful care management program. The critical steps of patient identification and creation of specific disease interventions can be facilitated by using pharmacy encounter data, which are readily available to pharmacists. Pharmacists are uniquely positioned and trained to (1) optimize patient self-management skills by counseling patients, establishing medication compliance programs, and training patients in device utilization techniques and (2) serve as a pharmacotherapy expert to other health care providers. All of these skills and functions are necessary for the development and implementation of an effective disease management program. Pharmaceutical companies are encouraged to leverage utilization of pharmacists as valuable professionals who have the patient accessibility and pharmacotherapeutic expertise to facilitate establishment of practical and successful care management programs in the outpatient community. The resulting programs could then be used as marketing tools in disease-specific areas by the pharmaceutical industry.

REFERENCES

1. Armstrong EP, Langley PC. Disease management programs. Am J Health-Syst Pharm 1996;53:53-8.

2. Townsend RJ. Post-marketing drug research and development. Drug Intell Clin Pharm 1987;21:134-6.

3. Langley PC. Outcomes and modeling therapeutic interventions for economic evaluations. Clin Ther 1994;16:538-52.

4. Langley PC, Martin RE. Analytic and informational requirements in disease management proposals: a managed care perspective. J Pharm Technol 1997;13(Jan-Feb):15-20.

5. Sharkey SS, Tracy DM. Methods and tools for CPI. In: Horn SD, Hopkins DS, eds. Clinical practice improvement: a new technology for developing cost-effective quality health care. New York: Faulkner & Gray, 1994.

6. Langley PC, Langley-Hawthorne CE, Martin RE, Armstrong EP. Establishing the basis for successful disease management contracting. Am J Manage Care 1996; 2:1099-108.

7. Epstein RS, Sherwood LM. From outcomes research to disease management: a guide for the perplexed. Ann Intern Med 1996;124:832-7.

8. Martin RE. Designing an asthma disease management program in a managed care environment. Formulary 1997;32:269-78.

Pharmacists and Quality of Life Assessment

Matthew M. Murawski
John P. Bentley

INTRODUCTION

Open any basic marketing or marketing management text and you will find a reference to strategic management or strategic planning and acknowledgment of its importance in today's changing marketplace (1). A fundamental element in the strategic management process is environmental scanning, or the analysis of the external environment to determine opportunities and threats and of the environment internal to the organization to determine strengths and weaknesses (2). With respect to the external environment in which pharmaceutical marketers operate, there is little question that the current health care environment

Matthew M. Murawski, Ph.D., is Assistant Professor of Pharmacy Administration and Research Assistant Professor, Research Institute of Pharmaceutical Sciences, School of Pharmacy, University of Mississippi, University, MS 38677.

John P. Bentley, M.B.A., M.S., is Graduate Research Assistant, Research Institute of Pharmaceutical Sciences, and a graduate student in the Department of Pharmacy Administration, University of Mississippi.

A portion of this paper appeared in the article "Quality of Life: The New Pharmacokinetics," published in *Drug Topics* [1996;140(Aug):134] and is reprinted with permission from Medical Economics Co.

Dr. Murawski acknowledges support for this research in the form of a Pharmaceutical Research and Manufacturers of America Foundation 1997 Faculty Development Award in Pharmacoeconomics.

[Haworth co-indexing entry note]: "Pharmacists and Quality of Life Assessment." Murawski, Matthew M., and John P. Bentley. Co-published simultaneously in *Journal of Pharmaceutical Marketing Practice* (Pharmaceutical Products Press, an imprint of The Haworth Press, Inc.) Vol. 1, No. 2 (#2), 1998, pp. 81-115; and: *Marketing to Pharmacists: Understanding Their Role and Influence* (ed: Benjamin F. Banahan III) Pharmaceutical Products Press, an imprint of The Haworth Press, Inc., 1998, pp. 81-115. Single or multiple copies of this article are available for a fee from The Haworth Document Delivery Service [1-800-342-9678, 9:00 a.m. - 5:00 p.m. (EST). E-mail address: getinfo@haworthpressinc.com].

contains numerous and diverse variables that may be classified as opportunities and/or threats. While not all of these variables are under the direct control of the marketing department or the organization as a whole, it is worthwhile to have an appreciation and understanding for these variables, as they can have an effect on the long-term operations of the firm. One such variable operating in the pharmaceutical marketer's external environment is the pharmacist's role and involvement in quality of life assessment. On the surface, this activity appears to be a threat for pharmaceutical marketers. However, an understanding of the issues underlying this growing role for pharmacists may lead to an opportunity for a win-win-win situation for the pharmacy practitioner, the pharmaceutical marketer, and most importantly, the patient.

The purpose of this article is to provide the pharmaceutical marketer with an introduction to the role of the pharmacist in quality of life assessment and many of the issues that are related to the undertaking of such a role. To achieve this, the article is divided into six sections. The first section will provide necessary background about the changes in the health care system underlying the growing use of quality of life measures and the evolution of the practice of pharmacy relative to quality of life. A discussion concerning the conceptualization of quality of life and the applications of quality of life measures will then be presented. The third section will focus on applying quality of life in pharmacy. Issues involved in measuring quality of life in the pharmacy setting will then be discussed. Data concerning pharmacists' knowledge base regarding quality of life and their perceptions of the construct will then be presented. Finally, the paper will conclude with a discussion of the impact of the role of the pharmacist in quality of life assessment on the practices of the pharmaceutical marketer.

BACKGROUND

Changes in the Health Care System Underlying the Growing Use of Quality of Life Measures

Several authors have offered discussions concerning the traditional model of medical decision making (i.e., the clinical paradigm) (3-6). These authors note that the clinical paradigm, or the biomedical model, has as its focus mechanism, causation, pathological processes, biophysiological variables, and clinical outcomes (3). As a result, "traditional medical decision making focuses on clinical indicators of disease and [clinical] outcomes" (5). While clinical indicators (e.g., blood pressure, serum cholesterol) and clinical outcomes (e.g., stroke, heart attack, death) are quantifiable and generally accepted and understood by practitioners, the definition of health inherent in the biomedical model is narrow, focusing on the function of organs and cells rather than on the function of individuals (4, 5). Many times the variables assessed in the traditional clinical paradigm are not as relevant to patients as variables such as functioning and well being. Wilson and Kaplan note that "perhaps the strongest indictment of the biomedical model is that it often does not meet the needs of patients" (4).

In addition to the limitations associated with the traditional medical decision-making model, several factors in recent years have led the health care community to consider additional measures of health and outcomes of medical decision making. One significant factor may be the result of the success of medical science. At the turn of the century, most patient deaths were the result of acute or infectious disease states. As a result of the progress in treating such disease conditions, many of the challenges that remain involve the treatment of chronic, often incurable diseases (7-10). In the evaluation of treatment alternatives for disease states that are often terminal, improvement in mortality is the outcome measure of primary importance. However, when treating chronic disease states, for which mortality is less of an issue, the adverse effects of therapy become more important relative to the disease. These adverse effects are experienced for a longer time and have a greater impact on patient compliance. Consequently, traditional measures of mortality or physiologic status appear limited in judging the benefits and risks associated with treatment of chronic conditions, while there is a growing need for means to measure functional status and HRQOL (11-16).

Other possible factors that contribute to the interest in using additional measures of health and outcomes for assessing medical decision making include: high and growing expenditures, incomplete health care coverage of individuals, growing concern over the value received for each health care dollar, pressures for technology assessment, development of practice guidelines, growing concern for patient preferences and autonomy, changes in the patient population itself, and a continued emphasis on health promotion and disease prevention

(17-25). Additionally, Greenfield and Nelson note that the traditional measures in health care are increasingly seen to be insufficient by themselves for two reasons: they fail to encompass other dimensions of health, such as social and mental aspects, and they are not universally relevant to all patients with a given disease or problem (23). The traditional, physiologic measures used to measure the impact of chronic disease "provide information to clinicians, but are of limited use to the patient; they often correlate poorly with functional capacity and well-being, the areas in which patients are most interested and most familiar" (26).

Kozma, Reeder, and Schulz have summarized the situation by noting that several medical, ethical, and societal issues are forcing health care practitioners to consider a more comprehensive model for medical decision making (5). In an effort to incorporate other measures of health and outcomes into the medical decision-making process in addition to the traditional clinical and biophysiological variables of the biomedical model, these authors developed the Economic, Clinical, and Humanistic Outcomes (ECHO) model. The ECHO model is a useful framework for examining the outcomes of medical care interventions (e.g., treatment with pharmaceutical products and services) and reminds us that the value of a pharmaceutical product or service is determined by "a combination of traditional clinical-based outcomes [and] more contemporary measures of economic efficiency and quality" rather than by reliance on any one particular outcome (5). Thus, humanistic outcomes, such as the impact of treatment and/or disease on a patient's quality of life, can be as important as clinical outcomes or economic outcomes in evaluating the value of a treatment alternative. However, the ECHO model calls for more than a subjective, nonspecific assessment of humanistic outcomes; the focus with respect to humanistic data is on systematic collection to assess value (5). The importance of standardized, systematic collection of humanistic data is demonstrated by observing the results of studies that show health care practitioners (typically physicians) are often poor and inaccurate judges of patient functioning and quality of life (27-29).

The Evolution of the Practice of Pharmacy Relative to Quality of Life

Given that changes in the health care environment and the recognition of the problems associated with relying solely on the traditional biomedical model are causing an increased emphasis to be placed on humanistic outcomes such as quality of life, what has happened in the evolutionary path of pharmacy with respect to quality of life? Today, the profession of pharmacy continues its evolution from a primary role of dispensing prefabricated drug products to a more encompassing mission of "serving society as the profession responsible for the appropriate use of medications, devices, and services to achieve optimal therapeutic outcomes" (30). Pharmacists are increasingly being asked to take responsibility for patients' health outcomes, including quality of life (6).

No discussion of the evolution of pharmacy with respect to quality of life would be complete without an analysis of the definition of pharmaceutical care provided by Hepler and Strand: "the responsible provision of drug therapy for the purpose of achieving definite outcomes that improve a patient's quality of life" (31). Of course, quality of life in this definition is more in the manner of an idealistic absolute, an aspiration of practice rather than a reference to formalized, structured quality of life measurement. Nevertheless, it does establish a framework in which such measurement becomes relevant to pharmacy practice.

Both the APhA mission statement for pharmacy and the concept of pharmaceutical care as formulated by Hepler and Strand focus on the pharmacist's responsibility for therapeutic outcomes. Reeder has suggested that "in a reformed health care system, pharmacists must assume responsibility for the humanistic, clinical, and economic outcomes of pharmaceutical therapy" (32). Specific to the pharmacist's responsibility for humanistic outcomes, Osterhaus and Osterhaus, both community pharmacists, state that, "since drug therapy plays such an important role in establishing and maintaining patients' quality of life, we must expand our professional roles to include the use of quality of life survey data if we are to adequately monitor our clients' progress and response to therapy" (33).

In its Statement on Pharmaceutical Care, the American Society of Health-System Pharmacists (ASHP) states:

> Some tools exist now for assessing a patient's quality of life. These tools are still evolving, and pharmacists should maintain familiarity with the literature on this subject. A complete assessment of a patient's quality of life should include both objective

and subjective (e.g., the patient's own) assessments. Patients should be involved, in an informed way, in establishing quality of life goals for their therapies. (34)

The ASHP statement raises the issue that pharmacists need to be knowledgeable about quality of life and its measurement: as a competency or skill associated with practice. If the goal of the care provided by pharmacists is to improve a patient's quality of life, pharmacists need the ability to document the quality of life of their patients.

The previous discussion demonstrates that the evolving role of the profession of pharmacy calls for its practitioners to embrace the concept of quality of life. Because of their consistent contact with patients, pharmacists appear to be in an ideal position to collect and use quality of life information in their practice. It has been suggested that pharmacists "are already experienced at helping patients maintain or improve their quality of life within the context of their medical treatment" (35). In fact, most would agree that health care practitioners, including pharmacists, have always incorporated humanistic outcomes into the traditional model of their practice in a subjective, nonspecific manner (5). Over 65% of the respondents to a survey of community pharmacies replied that they attempt to assess the health-related quality of life of their patients; however, most respondents who reportedly assess the heath-related quality of life of their patients use subjective criteria (general discussion with patients) rather than objective criteria (having patients complete multiple choice questionnaires concerning their HRQOL) (36). Questions such as, "How are you?" and, "Are you better, the same, or worse than the last time I saw you?" are fairly common in practice (37). However, this type of data collection is nonsystematic, anecdotal, and unidimensional. It does not allow for quantification, nor does it allow the practitioner to objectively assess the impact of disease and treatment on quality of life. Finally, as will be discussed in a subsequent section, such an approach fails to assess the multidimensionality of a patient's quality of life. A more systematic approach to the collection of data is required, and there are currently several instruments available that are suitable for such an approach.

Interestingly, lack of patient information and limited access to pertinent medical information have been cited in the literature as barriers to the delivery of clinical services and pharmaceutical care (38-42). Systematic collection of quality of life data as offered by many currently available instruments offers pharmacists a method of generating their own patient-specific information.

It appears that quality of life considerations are not only growing in their importance in the delivery of health care but are also a part of the delivery of pharmaceutical care. Pharmaceutical marketers need to understand the role of pharmacists with respect to quality of life. If nothing else, quality of life implications of drug therapy can produce meaningful effects with respect to profitability. For example, Jack calculated that claims of positive impact on patient quality of life resulted in an increase in sales of captopril in the range of $375 million (43). This certainly suggests that patients and practitioners are receptive to the idea of providing pharmaceutical therapy in such a way that patient quality of life is maximized and that this receptiveness is reflected in the marketplace. However, the promotion of positive drug effects on patient quality of life and its subsequent impact on sales is not the only aspect of quality of life and the pharmacist that is important for the pharmaceutical marketer to understand. Pharmacists may act as disseminators of quality of life information available for pharmaceutical products (44). Furthermore, as will be described in subsequent sections, pharmacists may be able to use quality of life instruments in their practices to detect medication-related problems and communicate these problems to prescribers, to evaluate and monitor drug therapy, to screen for functional deficiencies in their patients and refer these patients to other health professionals, and to document the effects of their interventions on patients' quality of life. In essence, pharmacy practitioners may use this information in conjunction with physicians to initiate and modify drug therapy. Understanding the role of the pharmacist with respect to patient quality of life is certainly necessary to be able to accurately assess all aspects of the pharmaceutical marketer's external environment.

Angaran has noted that "[quality of life] may be the new pharmacokinetics in its importance to the profession and our patients" (45). The use of the term pharmacokinetics in such a context suggests a much different, more immediate relationship between the practice of pharmacy and quality of life measurement than the abstract definition of pharmaceutical care or the marketing of pharmaceuticals. It is this level of application–involving quality of life measurement in direct patient care–that this article explores. However, to allow the pharmaceutical marketer to appreciate the utility of quality of life measurement to pharmacy and its potential applications, it is first necessary to explore what is meant by the terms quality of life (QOL) and health-related quality of life (HRQOL) and the general applications of measures of these constructs.

QUALITY OF LIFE AND ITS APPLICATIONS

What Constitutes Quality of Life?

A key factor in understanding quality of life measurement as it applies to pharmacy practice is the concept of multiple dimensions of quality of life. Quality of life is made up of a number of different dimensions (or as they are sometimes referred to, domains), and each contributes to the individual's perception of overall life quality. So while it may not be possible to directly measure an individual's estimate of his/her current life quality, it may be possible to measure levels of the various components that the majority of people use to derive their estimate.

Quality of life as an overall assessment of well being is commonly thought to be made up of at least the dimensions of physical status, psychological status, social interactions, economic status (including vocation and housing), and spiritual or religious status (46). Some researchers include other dimensions, but these five constitute the core domains of quality of life for which consensus exists.

Of course, not all of these dimensions are subject to alteration in response to some interventions or are particularly relevant to some areas of study. As an example, it is hard to imagine how two different compounds used to treat hypertension would differ in their impact on spirituality or housing. Additionally, these dimensions may be quite difficult to measure in any sort of objective manner. To resolve these difficulties, many researchers utilize the concept of health-related quality of life (HRQOL). HRQOL is conceptualized as those aspects of quality of life directly affected by a patient's health. By restricting the definition in this manner, it is possible to avoid some of the thorny measurement issues and to produce measures that are relevant and responsive to changes in a patient's health status typical of health care interventions or normal disease progression. While the component dimensions of HRQOL, like those of QOL, continue to be debated and refined, dimensions that are commonly included in the construct include physical functioning, psychological functioning, social functioning, cognitive functioning, and general well-being. Within each of the broad component dimensions are subcomponents (47). Thus, the physical functioning dimension may include measurements of mobility, bodily pain, activities of daily living, and sleep. The social functioning dimension may include interpersonal contacts, quantity and quality of social ties, freedom from limitations in the performance of usual roles, and recreation. The psychological functioning dimension may include measures of anxiety/depression and behavioral/emotional control.

Of course, it can be argued that treatments provided in the health care realm can and do alter individuals' satisfaction with QOL dimensions that are not commonly included in definitions of HRQOL. As an example, the individual suffering from a wasting disease may be forced to reassess employment opportunities if cure or mitigation of the disease process does not occur. This is a case where the provision of health care services clearly does affect dimensions of QOL not commonly included in HRQOL. The problem, from the scientist's point of view, is that so many other factors not relevant to the provision of health care services may also be responsible for changes in the patient's employment status. Employment status may change in response to economic conditions, patient choice, or acts of God. Inclusion of this and similar dimensions in QOL measurement when applied in health services research may result in the detection of changes in these dimensions, but it becomes difficult, if not impossible, to establish whether these observed changes are the consequence of the provision of health care services. These tenuous, sometimes spurious, associations between medical treatment and patient status in certain dimensions can be eliminated by limiting the definition of QOL to those dimensions that are clearly related to patient health status–hence, HRQOL. The result is measurement instruments that are of far more relevance and practical value to the researcher and the practitioner.

Uses and Applications of Health-Related Quality of Life Measures

The development of HRQOL measurement instruments is usually thought to have begun as early as the 1940's with the Karnofsky Performance Status instrument, a practitioner-completed scale of patient functional status. Serious development efforts resulting in the production of what are recognized today as HRQOL instruments began in the 1970's. As the development of HRQOL instruments has progressed, a great many different uses for these instruments have been suggested (Table 1) (48-53).

The methodological framework for the development and assessment of health status measures described by Kirshner and Guyatt emphasizes the specific purposes for which an instrument will be used (54). These purposes (discrimination, prediction, and evaluation) serve to clarify issues related to the construction and validation of quality of life measures. Related to these purposes, Ware has defined four pressing applications of health surveys containing measures of patient functioning and well-being (55). The first application is health care policy studies to evaluate alternatives for organizing and financing health care services. Policy makers and the public are beginning to demand information about the effects of different cost-containment strategies on patient health outcomes. The Health Insurance Experiment (HIE) and the Medical Outcomes Study (MOS) of the 1970's and 1980's are examples. As Ware points out, "the MOS was designed specifically to explore the effects of cost containment on patient outcomes, including a broad array of outcomes from the patient's point of view" (55).

The second pressing application is clinical trials of new interventions and technology. As alluded to earlier, several factors have forced the medical community to consider variables other than the traditional clinical indicators when evaluating therapy. It is becoming more accepted that treatment alternatives and health care technologies "should be evaluated in terms of their impact on patient functioning and well-being in addition to traditionally defined medical endpoints and their dollar costs" (55).

TABLE 1. General Uses of HRQOL Measurement Instruments.

- Measuring the effectiveness of interventions
- Selecting treatments/making clinical decisions at the patient level
- Assessing the quality of care
- Detecting disease and dysfunction
- Assessing the extent of disease and dysfunction
- Estimating the needs of the population/community resources
- Understanding the causes and consequences of differences in health
- As an adjunct in the training of physicians

The third application of health surveys is in the monitoring of the health of the general population. Traditional measures do not reveal much information about the health of the population. Population mortality statistics tell little about the health of the general population in well-developed countries. Standardized measures of health status could be used to monitor the health of the general population.

The fourth application is clinical decision making in medical practice. Ware comments that standardized health surveys have the potential to become the new "laboratory tests" of medical practice (55). Currently, however, these surveys are not being used in the clinical setting to any great extent. At best, functioning and well-being are discussed informally during the patient history.

With respect to the use of health status measures for clinical decision making in medical practice, Greenfield and Nelson propose three major applications (23). The first of these clinical uses is the description of the natural history of disease and the impact of the disease on health status. This application has advanced the basic knowledge of disease progression and aging. It has demonstrated how diseases such as heart disease, diabetes, and depression can influence health status. This application began opening the eyes of the medical community to health status and quality of life assessment.

The second application is the evaluation of treatment and its effectiveness. This application is related to Ware's second use of health status measures, clinical trials of new interventions and technologies. Information about the clinical trial is disseminated to the medical community. Like any other information generated from a clinical trial, health status information now has the potential to influence caregiving decisions. In this application, assessment of HRQOL is a clinical trial outcome and still takes place at the population level. However, data on the impact of specific treatments on HRQOL is now available.

The third use of health status measures in clinical settings is measuring quality of care at the individual patient level. According to Greenfield and Nelson, this use has the greatest potential for affecting day-to-day clinical practice (23). This approach is not a research approach, as the other two applications are, but a practical application. This application would require the collection and interpretation of health related quality of life information from patients. Recently, there has been a growing interest in the implementation of routine quality of life assessment in the clinical setting through the collection and use of

HRQOL information for individual patient assessment and treatment monitoring (21, 56-65). Deyo and Carter suggest that health status measures could be used for a variety of purposes in clinical settings, including "screening for functional problems, monitoring disease progression or therapeutic response, improving doctor-patient communications, assessing the quality of care, and providing case-mix adjustment for comparing other outcomes between patient groups" (66).

A number of outpatient randomized controlled trials have been conducted in which health status information about patients was provided to one group of physicians (experimental group) but not to a control group of physicians (67-71). The research generally demonstrates that physicians report that health status information has some clinical utility; however, very few studies have been able to demonstrate any significant objective benefits (e.g., improved health status reports of patients, better compliance, more satisfaction with care) as a consequence of providing this information to physicians.

Measures of functional assessment have been integrated into some aspects of clinical practice, such as geriatrics, rheumatology, and psychiatry. While the literature on the effectiveness of clinical HRQOL assessment is limited, evidence has been presented that comprehensive geriatric assessment (quantification of all relevant medical, functional, and psychosocial attributes and deficits) is effective in the care of the elderly (72). The American College of Physicians has issued a position paper urging the evaluation of health status in the routine management of older adults (73). This paper states that, "although no single test is universally recommended, selection of a comprehensive screen followed by a group of targeted instruments can be useful in systematically assessing functional deficits that otherwise might be overlooked by conventional examination methods" (73).

A number of reasons have been proposed as to why significant objective benefits of HRQOL assessment in the general clinical setting fail to be demonstrated. Rubenstein et al. propose that physicians may not be the appropriate change agents to whom interventions should be targeted (69). The authors suggest that patients or other allied health professionals might be better candidates for intervention. Although Rubenstein et al. do not specifically mention the pharmacist as a collector and user of heath-related quality of life information, other authors have alluded to this role. For example, MacKeigan and Pathak suggest that "a brief QOL questionnaire could feasibly be completed along with every medication history conducted by the pharmacist" (74). The information provided by this quality of life assessment may assist pharmacists in the detection of drug-related problems and may also be a useful way to quantitatively track patient progress toward therapeutic goals in certain chronic disease states (74). Salek suggests that "pharmacy practitioners could measure the impact of the disease and treatment on a patient's quality of life as a routine assessment by using one of the existing instruments (questionnaire) which has proved to be valid and reliable" (44).

APPLYING HRQOL IN PHARMACY

There appears to be a role for pharmacy practitioners in quality of life assessment, and quality of life considerations are growing in their importance with respect to the delivery of pharmaceutical care. The pharmacist's role may be that of a disseminator of quality of life information at the individual level in the management of patients or at more general practice-based or population-based levels. This section will explore some of these roles in greater detail and will address how HRQOL can be applied in pharmacy. Before examining these applications, the first part of this section will analyze the parallel between measurement strategies used in HRQOL assessment and the multidimensional changes in health status produced by pharmaceutical services.

Multiple Dimensions of HRQOL and Pharmacy

There is one facet of HRQOL measurement in particular that merits further discussion, specifically, the serendipitous alignment between the measurement strategies developed for HRQOL and the nature of the changes in patient status characteristic of the provision of pharmaceutical services. It is the nature of the relationship between measurement and practice that makes HRQOL technology of such great potential importance to pharmacy.

What is the nature of this congruence between pharmaceutical services and HRQOL measurement? Consider the likely outcomes of the provision of pharmaceutical services, including the effects of specific products, the provision of specific services, and the provision of general services. Ideally, in the case of a specific product, there are improvements in the target disease or the target symptoms for which the product has been prescribed. In the provision of specific services such as anticoagulation consults, the ideal outcome is optimization of therapy for a particular product such as warfarin. The ideal outcome of the provision of general pharmaceutical services is similar except that the focus of general services is not limited to a narrow component of the patient's therapy.

Each level of care is focused on achieving particular therapeutic goals. An important question is how to measure how effectively these therapeutic goals are reached at each level of service. For the individual product, the primary outcome measure is most likely the level of the relevant target symptom. Thus, an antihypertensive product is often evaluated in terms of its ability to decrease patient blood pressure (75). For the provision of specific services, the primary outcome measure is likely to be that benefit which led to the specific service being provided in the first place. For the case of the warfarin consult, the benefit may be a lower incidence of thrombolytic occlusions. Unfortunately, it is extremely difficult to identify such a primary outcome measure for the provision of general pharmacy services. Because in day-to-day practice the pharmacist may intervene in any area of the patient's therapy, with a nearly infinite number of possible benefits, formalized assessment of the effectiveness of such services becomes extremely difficult. One approximation that has been used in the past is the incidence of adverse reactions (consequences) in the patient population base. Problems with the use of this measure as a primary outcome indicator are that it only reflects negative results, the incidence in most populations is low, and accurate definition and detection of adverse reactions can be quite difficult.

However, the use of the incidence of adverse reactions as an outcome measure illustrates the next point in this discussion. The provision of pharmaceutical services, at any level, is never without consequences of some kind. For the individual product, a positive therapeutic effect on the target symptom is in almost every case associated with some negative consequence for the patient. An antibiotic may cause diarrhea, an ACE inhibitor may cause cough, and reserpine may cause depression. In each of these examples, the adverse consequence is divorced functionally from the positive benefit for which the medication has been prescribed. In fact, for the examples of reserpine and ACE inhibitors, the link between the use of the product and the adverse consequence was not immediately apparent. This is not surprising when one considers that most measures used to assess the efficacy of these products would, by their nature, be restricted in scope to the product's action on the target disease or symptom.

Of course, the structure of clinical trials is such that many of the adverse consequences of a product are identified in the preapproval process. But the difficulty of identification of negative and positive consequences of treatment increases by at least an order of magnitude when the next level, specific pharmaceutical services, is considered. In this case, there are not only the positive and negative consequences of a single medication involved. There is also the increased danger that may be associated with the provision of the service. Using the example of anticoagulation consults for warfarin, a subtherapeutic dosage level may have left the patient at risk for vascular incidents. Attainment of an appropriate dosage level may reduce the probability of vascular or coronary occlusion, but it also increases the likelihood of hemorrhagic crises. Another confounding factor that increases the complexity of assessment at this level is the interaction of the target medication with other medications. In the same manner that the adverse consequences of use of a specific medication may manifest themselves functionally separate from the target effect, drug-drug interactions can produce effects remote from the therapeutic actions of the drugs involved.

When the level of general pharmaceutical services is considered, the complexities of identification and measurement increase exponentially. Not only are all the confounding factors of specific pharmaceutical services present, but the possible actions and interactions are no longer limited by a specific target drug. The possible number of positive or negative effects on patient status rapidly approach infinity. The difficulties inherent in attempting to measure a pharmacist's impact on patient health in this morass of variables may explain why research data on the benefits of general pharmacy services are so hard to come by.

There is, however, another way to conceptualize the problem. The positive and negative responses to therapy have, up to this point in the discussion, been presented as occurring in some cases in different bodily systems or as being functionally separate from the target effect for which the medication or service has been provided. Another useful way to conceptualize this separation between therapeutic target effect and associated positive or negative consequences is to think of the different biochemical level changes produced by pharmaceutical services being reflected in changes in different dimensions of HRQOL.

This is the key to understanding why HRQOL measurement can be of such value to pharmacy. In other disciplines, the primary advantage of using HRQOL measurement is that the instruments are thought to express the impact of care from the patient's perspective or in terms of the patient's experience (76-78). As an example, sedimentation rate has been used for some time as a laboratory indicator of the severity of rheumatoid arthritis, so the drug development process favors products or therapies that produce the desired changes in sedimentation rate (79). But do changes in the sedimentation rate result in changes in the patient's experience of the disease state? Do medications that produce changes in this laboratory test also produce changes in the patient's HRQOL? The ability of HRQOL measurements to detect differences in patient status in HRQOL dimensions other than the dimension for which the therapy is targeted is a recognized but secondary benefit.

For pharmacy, the ability of HRQOL measurement to detect therapeutically remote differences in patient status is of special utility, since perhaps more than in any other discipline, the effects of pharmacy services manifest themselves across different HRQOL dimensions. Put another way, what is it that pharmacists do? The concept of pharmaceutical care suggests that what they do is to optimize pharmaceutical therapy. How do you tell if pharmaceutical therapy is optimized or not? You examine and quantify all the various and sundry possible impacts on patient status that may or may not occur with the infinite combinations of therapeutic alternatives that may be prescribed and then begin to explore the relative tradeoffs associated with all the possible alternatives that could be used to achieve the therapeutic goals for a given patient, or you could measure the patient's HRQOL as you try each of the available alternatives.

In the deliberate and considered world of academic research, it is possible (yet quite difficult) to isolate a small part of the complex picture of pharmaceutical services, identify all relevant outcomes, and begin to assess the pharmacist's impact on patient status. What makes the use of HRQOL measurement so exciting is that this technology is rapidly becoming compact and easy enough to administer that it can be applied directly in the pharmacy and to the individual patient. The individual pharmacist may have for years advised and educated patients and practitioners about minor changes in therapy that the pharmacist felt would benefit the patient, given the pharmacist's special knowledge of the patient's concerns and the intricacies of the relevant product's therapeutic effects, side effects, and interactions with the rest of the patient's therapy. HRQOL measurement at long last provides a tool for measuring the benefits of such "tinkering" and does so in such a manner that it can be used at the community pharmacy level.

Applications of HRQOL in Pharmacy

Given the unique suitability of HRQOL measurement to pharmacy, there are a number of possible applications of this technology within the profession. These can be categorized according to the four *P*'s–product, patient, pharmacist, and population.

Product Applications

Product applications of HRQOL are perhaps the most remote from the individual pharmacy or pharmacist. With the possible exception of large teaching institutions, product evaluation is not likely to occur at the individual pharmacy level, rather, the pharmacist will need a solid knowledge base regarding HRQOL measurement to evaluate available product information provided by manufacturers and/or researchers when considering that product for inclusion on the formulary or for addition to a patient's therapy. Within this context, information on a product's impact on patient HRQOL can serve two purposes, assessment and comparison. When used as a means of assessment, HRQOL information tells the pharmacist what kind of changes in patient HRQOL are likely to be associated with this product. When used as a means of comparison, HRQOL information about two or more competing products can be evaluated to select the medication most likely to prove of maximum benefit for the pharmacist's individual patient or relevant patient population.

As a crude hypothetical example, two medications may be available that are equally efficacious in reaching a particular therapeutic goal. Drug X causes impairment of physical functioning, Drug Y impairment of cognitive functioning. The pharmacist, with his or her knowledge of the patient, may recommend use of Drug Y in a patient who earns a living as a construction worker, where physical functioning is at a premium. Drug X may be the best choice for a teacher or an accountant.

Patient Applications

Patient level use of HRQOL in pharmacy may be the most exciting application. The pharmacist can ask patients to complete a paper and pencil version of one of the available HRQOL instruments while waiting for prescriptions and then score the results manually. Another alternative would be to enter the results into one of the currently available software packages that incorporate automatic scoring, assessment, and record keeping of the patient's HRQOL information. In the future, the pharmacist will have the third alternative of having the patient complete the HRQOL instrument using computer-assisted technology, where the patient enters responses directly into a simplified keyboard and the data are immediately recorded, scored, and compared with the patient's previously recorded information.

However the HRQOL data are obtained, the pharmacist can then use the information for two purposes: diagnosis and monitoring. As pharmacists gain familiarity with HRQOL data, it may become possible for the practitioner to examine patient scores and identify characteristic patterns of HRQOL that indicate therapeutic problems. The monitoring function comes into play when changes in therapy are initiated, at which time repeated measurements of patient HRQOL will allow the pharmacist to assess the extent to which the new therapeutic strategy is effective (80, 81).

Pharmacist Applications

The next category of HRQOL application is the pharmacist. If the practice of pharmacy is moving toward a patient-centered model, wherein the pharmacist's responsibility is to ensure that pharmaceutical therapy for the individual patient has been optimized as much as possible, then it stands to reason that pharmacists will differ in their ability to accomplish this goal. As an illustrative contrast, in the dispensing centered model, there was little or nothing to differentiate the superlative pill counter from the mediocre one. In a patient-centered model, however, the variance in pharmacists' ability to improve patient outcomes does permit differing levels of pharmacist ability to become evident, and patient HRQOL data may be used as an indicator of a pharmacist's proficiency and skill.

Thus, records of accumulated patient response to an individual pharmacist's intervention may be examined when the pharmacist is considered for hiring or promotion; demonstrated ability to influence patient HRQOL positively may become a requirement for third-party reimbursement; and evidence of positive impact on patient HRQOL may become the grounds for premium reimbursement schemes. While many pharmacists would greet the use of HRQOL information in such a manner less than enthusiastically, using HRQOL data as an indicator of pharmacist ability is not by any means all bad. Recall that in the past there was little that differentiated one pharmacist (or pharmacy) from another. Pharmacy as a profession was almost forced to compete purely on the basis of price. Imagine the differences in the pharmacy marketplace if pharmacists and pharmacies competed on the basis of knowledge, skill, and dedication.

Population Applications

The final category of HRQOL application for pharmacy is at the level of the population. HRQOL instruments have already been used to document the prevalence of various degrees of impairment in study populations. In fact, this application is one for which many instruments were first designed (82). To understand one way this type of application may be of use to pharmacists, it is first necessary to consider the reimbursement environment. Many third-party payers are moving toward some form of managed care, as are public payers such as Medicaid. At the heart of the managed care approach is the idea of risk sharing between the payer and the provider. This is usually operationalized in some type of capitation arrangement. In a capitation reimbursement system, the provider agrees to provide services to x number of patients for a given year. In return, the payer agrees to pay a specified dollar amount per patient per month (PMPM). If the provider is able to provide all agreed-upon services for less than the PMPM reimbursement, a profit is realized. If costs exceed the PMPM, then the provider loses money. The provider must continue to provide these services or be in breach of contract. Thus, the payer shares the risk with the provider. The payer is being paid a certain PMPM amount for providing all health care services, and the provider gets a piece of that pie. If for some reason health care costs increase dramatically in the population, then both the provider and the payer may end up losing money.

Of course, it is hard for a single pharmacy, or even a relatively large pharmacy chain, to equal the predictive expertise of a large health maintenance organization in these matters. In these cases, the pharmacy may end up carrying a little more of the risk than might be ideal, mostly due to a relative lack of information regarding the health status of the patients in question. HRQOL information, gathered and sorted according to coverage, may be a means by which pharmacists can make more informed decisions about reimbursement suitability when considering which contracts to accept and which to reject. Thus, HRQOL may be used for risk assessment at the population level.

In the same way, the pharmacist may use the accumulated HRQOL information from the patient base to identify the prevalence of problems in the population being served. This application–needs assessment–allows the pharmacist to identify those services for which the greatest demand exists in the patient population. With knowledge of the needs of the population, the pharmacist or pharmacy can ensure provision of the expertise or services that will prove most beneficial to patients and the bottom line. The pharmacy applications are summarized in Table 2.

MEASURING HRQOL IN THE PHARMACY SETTING

A complete review of the measurement process with respect to quality of life is beyond the scope of this article. The reader is referred to several review articles and books that provide a good background in

TABLE 2. Pharmacy Applications of HRQOL Instruments.

Product
- Assessment
- Comparison

Patient
- Diagnosis
- Monitoring

Pharmacist
- Reimbursement
- Differentiating Providers

Population
- Risk Assessment
- Needs Assessment

HRQOL assessment (26, 74, 83-90). Because a major portion of this article has been devoted to pharmacists' involvement in quality of life measurement in direct patient care, several measurement issues relevant to such an undertaking warrant further discussion. These issues include the availability, length, and measurement properties of HRQOL instruments.

Availability of HRQOL Measurement Instruments

The first issue to consider is the availability of measurement instruments. There are a number of existing quality of life instruments available that may be considered for testing in the clinical setting (63). Bungay and Wagner note that quality of life "questionnaires are mature enough for use in clinical practice and now require evaluation in patient care settings by clinicians" (91). Several measures have been designed for individual patient use in routine clinical practice. The Dartmouth COOP Poster Charts and the Functional Status Questionnaire are examples (56, 92). Other surveys were designed for group-level applications but have been recommended for use in clinical practice. Examples of these instruments include the Nottingham Health Profile, the Duke Health Profile (The DUKE), and the SF-36 Health Survey (93-97).

Length of HRQOL Measurement Instruments

A significant barrier to using patient assessments as outcome measures in direct patient care is lack of time (98). Hence, a characteristic of HRQOL instruments that is especially salient to applications in pharmacy is length. Instruments differ in the number of items they use to sample the various dimensions of HRQOL. Longer instruments take more time to complete and thus create a greater respondent burden, as well as incur greater costs in printing, administration, and scoring. The tradeoff is that longer instruments, as a generalization, provide a more precise description of the respondent's HRQOL status. The relationship is roughly analogous to the trade-off between speed and resolution for photographic emulsions. For high-resolution applications such as research, longer instruments are usually preferred. In most population monitoring applications a shorter instrument will be adequate. In response to the different needs of potential users, instrument developers are beginning to provide different length versions of their instruments. A good example of this is the Quality of Life in Epilepsy (QOLIE) inventory, developed jointly by RAND and Professional Postgraduate Services. This instrument is available in 10-, 31-, and 89-item versions (99, 100).

Short, generic instruments that could be used for general population screening include the Medical Outcomes Trust Short Form 36- or 12-item instruments (the SF-36 and the SF-12), the Health Outcomes Institute's 39- and 12-item Health Status Questionnaires (the HSQ-39 and the HSQ-12), and the 17-item Duke Health Profile (94, 97, 101-103). The Duke Health Profile is an example of a short generic instrument. While taking only a few minutes for the average patient to complete, the single-page Duke Health Profile provides 11 subscale scores. These are physical health, mental health, social health, general health, perceived health, self-esteem, anxiety, depression, combined anxiety-depression, pain, and disability scores. The coding mechanism can be computerized, and a trained keypunch operator can enter approximately four instruments per minute. The Duke Health Profile is inexpensive to print, is inexpensive to mail, and provides an impressive amount of information for such a small package. The SF-12 is an even shorter instrument and, like the longer SF-36 from which it is derived, can be completed on scanable sheets that can be fed into a scanning machine immediately and scored within a few seconds. While the hardware required for this high-speed processing is somewhat expensive, high-volume applications make its use worthwhile, and if instrument use at the pharmacy level becomes common, economies of scale are likely to bring down initial costs for automatic scanning equipment considerably.

The patient can now complete an HRQOL instrument using computer-assisted technology. The patient enters responses directly into a simplified keyboard or onto a touch screen and the data are immediately recorded, scored, and compared with the patient's previously recorded information. One company, Assist Technologies, currently offers an outcomes software package that allows patients to enter responses to almost any quality of life questionnaire directly into the computer by touching the computer screen.

Pharmacists may be concerned about patients' willingness to complete regular assessments of HRQOL. There is evidence in the literature that patients in general respond well to requests for completion of HRQOL instruments. This may be because the HRQOL instrument can be thought of as a formalized way of asking patients how they are doing, and most patients want their health care providers to have and to be interested in this information. Ultimately, though, the most salient determinant of patient acceptance of this technology will not be the time or effort required of the patient–it will be the extent to which the pharmacist uses the information it provides to interact with the patient and move toward optimal pharmaceutical therapy.

Measurement Properties of HRQOL Instruments

Another measurement issue relevant to pharmacists' involvement in quality of life assessment in direct patient care concerns the measurement properties of currently available instruments. The process involved in the development of an HRQOL instrument is quite complex and involved. In general, the instrument is examined to ensure that a sufficient number and type of items are included to assess all the relevant dimensions of interest, that these items display adequate variation from one patient to the next, that the instrument measures what it is meant to measure (the instrument's validity), that the instrument will measure the same level of HRQOL in a patient on two different occasions if the patient has not changed in any way (the instrument's test-retest reliability), and that the items in the instrument are correlated with one another (i.e., the items are homogeneous, that is, they measure the same concept) (the instrument's internal consistency reliability).

Without adequate information on an instrument's reliability and validity, the usefulness and interpretation of data obtained from an assessment instrument is subject to question. Furthermore, if an instrument is going to be used in the clinical setting for diagnostic purposes, information on sensitivity (the extent to which patients who have the characteristic are accurately classified) and specificity (the extent to which patients without the characteristic are accurately classified) is necessary (i.e., the instrument's discriminating power). If the instrument is to be used for monitoring patients over time, the responsiveness (the ability of the instrument to detect change) of the instrument becomes a critical factor.

To be used for individual patient level applications, a scale generally has to meet more stringent standards for reliability than it would for group level applications. For example, instruments which are used to make clinical decisions about individual patients require reliability scores between 0.90 and 0.95, whereas instruments used at the group level require somewhat lower reliability scores (around 0.70) (104). Reliability of the instrument is an important consideration for individual-level applications because if "an unreliable instrument is used in the clinical setting, the clinician will not know if observed measurement differences are related to the patient's actual condition or to measurement artifact" (57).

With respect to measurement properties, McHorney and Tarlov reviewed five health status surveys that either were designed to be used in clinical practice or were designed for group-level applications but have been recommended for use in clinical practice (62). Taken as a whole, these instruments performed well with respect to practicality, breadth of health measured, the presence of floor effects (percentage of the sample achieving the worst possible score), and validity at the group level. However, significant ceiling effects (percentage of the sample achieving the best possible score) were found for most of the instruments, standards for reliability (both internal consistency and test-retest) were not met by any of the instruments, and evidence of validity at the individual patient level was lacking for most instruments. The authors concluded that the instruments reviewed may not be suitable for monitoring the health and treatment status of individual patients.

McHorney and Tarlov recognize that trade-offs exist between measurement simplicity and precision for individual patient level applications (62). Score distributions, reliability, and precision of an individual score favor longer measures, while ease of administration, low respondent burden, low costs of data collection and scoring, and ease of score interpretation favor briefer measures. They maintain that measurement precision should be the first priority in individual patient-level applications. However, Hays et al. suggest that "even if the measures fall short of the 0.90 reliability level, obtaining this information is preferred to not doing so. Although the confidence interval around an individual patient's score is wider than one might like, the interval is still tighter than that based on no information at all" (87).

McHorney and Tarlov offer for debate that their proposed standards may be too high (62). They cite several examples of commonly used clinical tests that fall short of the minimum standards of reliability for individual patient assessment. In a study of 24-hour test-retest reliabilities for blood pressure, the 0.90 standard for reliability was not met.

Systolic blood pressure and diastolic blood pressure reliabilities were 0.87 and 0.67, respectively (105). McHorney and Tarlov also note that some clinical tests have noteworthy floor and ceiling effects. However, the authors state that "clinicians do appear to develop an intuitive understanding of clinical test results that is shaped by years of formal medical education and clinical experience in interpreting scores in everyday patient care" (62). Applications of health status measures in clinical practice have been too few to date for clinicians to gain experience with these measures or to evaluate their utility.

The measurement properties of instruments are important considerations in the use of HRQOL measures at the individual patient level. While instrument standards have been proposed for this application, no such standards have been universally accepted (62). And while many instruments are available for evaluation in the clinical setting, there is currently very little clinical experience with the use of HRQOL measures, so it is very difficult, if not impossible, for health care practitioners to develop an intuitive understanding of the results. Clearly, such experience is needed. In addition, to meet clinical needs, it may be necessary to develop new instruments or adaptations of existing measures and scaling methods for individual-level assessment and monitoring (62).

PHARMACISTS AND QUALITY OF LIFE: WHERE DO THEY STAND?

Thus far, we have acknowledged that changes in the environment are causing quality of life considerations to grow in importance in the delivery of health care and in the delivery of pharmaceutical care. We have noted the parallel nature of measurement strategies used in HRQOL assessment and the multidimensional changes in health status produced by pharmaceutical services. We have outlined a number of potential applications of HRQOL in the pharmacy setting and discussed some measurement issues. The question that remains to be answered is where are pharmacists with respect to quality of life assessment? What are some of their general perceptions of quality of life? What is their knowledge base and familiarity with the concept? Are they willing to collect and use this information in their practice? What are the perceived barriers involved in such an undertaking?

Lindley and Hirsch have examined many of these questions with respect to oncology nurses (106). Their findings indicate that oncology "nurses value quality of life as an outcome measure of cancer treatment but lack knowledge regarding its measurability, particularly with respect to reliable tools and available time to assess it well" (106).

Bentley et al. have examined these issues with respect to community pharmacists (36). Community pharmacists' (n = 534) level of agreement with general attitudinal statements concerning quality of life can be found in Table 3. For this national sample of community pharmacists, HRQOL appears to be an important outcome of pharmaceutical care, consistent with Hepler and Strand's often-cited definition of pharmaceutical care (31). Additionally, pharmacists generally agree

TABLE 3. Pharmacist Agreement Ratings to Attitudinal Statements Concerning Quality of Life.

Item	Mean Response[a]
HRQOL is an important outcome of pharmaceutical care	5.9
Having information on a patient's HRQOL would assist me to provide better patient care	5.5
Pharmacists should assess their patient' HRQOL as part of their practice	4.9
HRQOL is a subjective and personal characteristic that cannot be measured, interpreted or compared	3.2
HRQOL is a term that was invented by the pharmaceutical industry to promote pharmaceuticals	2.6
Clinical measures, such as blood pressure or serum cholesterol, are more *quantifiable* than HRQOL information	5.6
Clinical measures, such as blood pressure or serum cholesterol, are more *easy to obtain* than HRQOL information	5.5
Clinical measures, such as blood pressure or serum cholesterol, are more *accurate* than HRQOL information	4.5
Clinical measures, such as blood pressure or serum cholesterol, are more *useful* measures than HRQOL	3.9
Clinical measures, such as blood pressure or serum cholesterol, are more *important* measures than HRQOL	3.9

[a]7-point scale, with 1 = strongly disagree and 7 = strongly agree

that having information on a patient's HRQOL would assist them in providing better patient care and that they should assess their patient's HRQOL as part of their practice. For the most part, pharmacists disagree that HRQOL is a personal characteristic that cannot be measured, interpreted, or compared, and they tend to have a greater level of disagreement that HRQOL was a term invented by the pharmaceutical industry to promote pharmaceuticals. This provides some evidence that pharmacists do not consider HRQOL data to be too "soft" for making decisions or view HRQOL is an unmeasurable construct. However, it is important to recognize that there are some pharmacists who do consider HRQOL to be unmeasurable, unquantifiable, or not as objective as other, traditional measures.

Pharmacists think that HRQOL information is less quantifiable than traditional clinical measures such as blood pressure measurement and serum cholesterol level. Additionally, pharmacists agreed that clinical measures are easier to obtain and, for the most part, more accurate than HRQOL information. However, there did not appear to be strong agreement that clinical measures were more useful or more important than HRQOL measures.

With respect to knowledge and familiarity, only slightly more than one-half of the respondents were familiar with the term and less than 5% were familiar with any formal HRQOL assessment instruments (36). The results also suggest that pharmacists who are familiar with the concept of HRQOL are most familiar with the colloquial use of the term rather than the more rigorous use of the term that has appeared in the health services and medical literature. Additionally, the self-reported knowledge of pharmacists concerning HRQOL was low, and respondents recognized a significant gap between their current knowledge and the level of knowledge needed to formally assess the HRQOL of their patients. While some pharmacists have a general understanding of HRQOL, it is likely that these pharmacists do not understand the nuances and methodologic concerns of formal quality of life assessment.

While recognizing their lack of preparation and training, community pharmacists appear to be willing to learn and use HRQOL assessment in their practices. After viewing examples of HRQOL measures (the Duke Health Profile and the QOLIE-10), over 80% of the respondents replied that a systematic approach to gathering information as provided by HRQOL instruments would be useful and over three-fourths expressed a willingness to use HRQOL instruments with their patients (36).

In addition to the educational barriers, community pharmacists recognized the difficulties in overcoming a number of other barriers and obstacles to measuring HRQOL in their practices. The barriers receiving the highest mean rating for the entire sample were lack of pharmacist time and the problems associated with storing and retrieving this information (36). Certainly the technology discussed earlier will be of great benefit in addressing the latter problem, but the former problem remains a significant barrier not only for HRQOL assessment but for pharmaceutical care in general. Addressing this barrier requires reworking the fundamental practices and responsibilities of the pharmacist.

Despite numerous obstacles, barriers, and unanswered questions (e.g., How can pharmacists use HRQOL information to help patients? Are current instruments adequate for use in the pharmacy setting at the individual patient level? Will pharmacist involvement in HRQOL assessment have an effect on economic, clinical, and humanistic outcomes?), pharmacists appear to have a somewhat favorable attitude toward the concept of HRQOL. While probably not large at this point, there is a segment of pharmacists who are innovative enough to become involved in the application of HRQOL in their practice settings. The following section will discuss the implications of this role for pharmaceutical marketers.

PHARMACEUTICAL MARKETERS
AND THE INVOLVEMENT OF PHARMACISTS
IN QUALITY OF LIFE ASSESSMENT

It is unlikely that every practicing community pharmacist will be assessing the HRQOL of patients tomorrow or even in the distant future. Nor is it likely that all pharmacists and pharmacies will be involved in the product, provider, or population applications discussed earlier. However, there is a great deal of potential for pharmacist involvement in many aspects of quality of life assessment and monitoring. In turn, the involvement of the pharmacist in this aspect of care has a considerable potential for affecting the external environment of the pharmaceutical marketer.

Marketers of pharmaceuticals need to be aware of the many uses and applications of HRQOL in pharmacy. Certainly pharmacists can act as disseminators of quality of life information as it relates to pharmaceutical products. They may act as a source of information for individual practitioners or at the institutional level. One or more pharmacists generally sit on the pharmacy and therapeutics committees of hospitals and managed care organizations. With quality of life considerations becoming more important in determining a drug's formulary status, pharmacists who are knowledgeable about quality of life issues can have a great deal of impact in these situations.

Related to this issue is the growing interest on the part of managed care organizations in the effectiveness of drug products (i.e., the drug effect in the "real world") as opposed to the efficacy of drug products (i.e., the drug effect in a tightly controlled clinical trial). HRQOL can be an important outcome variable in research that takes place in naturalistic settings, serving as a marker of effectiveness. The findings of such research have the potential to influence a drug's use in the managed care setting. The pharmacist can serve as a valuable source of information with respect to a drug's HRQOL effectiveness profile.

Beyond serving as a source of HRQOL information, pharmacy practitioners may use HRQOL data in conjunction with physicians to initiate and modify drug therapy. The potential impact of such activity on the sales of a pharmaceutical product can be quite large. Pharmacists come into contact with patients on a regular basis (perhaps more than any other health professional) and, if nothing else, pharmacists can serve as a source for data collection for postmarketing studies on the quality of life impact of pharmaceuticals.

Although there are a number of potential applications, pharmaceutical marketers also need to be aware that most pharmacists are not very familiar with the concept of HRQOL and the intricacies involved in its measurement. Pharmacist use of HRQOL information is still in the developmental stage. We believe the information presented here is a clear argument for the further development of HRQOL measurement in pharmacy. This suggests a continuing interest for the astute pharmaceutical marketer with respect to the pharmacist and quality of life. If pharmacists are moving down the path toward quality of life assessment, it should be the goal and aspiration of pharmaceutical marketers to ensure that such information be used in an appropriate manner. Pharmaceutical marketers can have a role not only in shaping pharmacy practitioners' education about and understanding of the effect of the marketers' products on quality of life but also in educating practitioners about quality of life in general. Pharmacists need education about the concept of HRQOL as well as about issues involved in its measurement. Furthermore, pharmacists need education about what they can do with HRQOL information and how it can be made relevant to their patients' welfare.

Salek suggests the following efforts to familiarize pharmacists with HRQOL and the importance of its measurement:

1. Increased involvement of professional organizations in providing information and increasing awareness
2. Incorporation of quality of life into undergraduate teaching programs
3. Organization of postgraduate continuing education programs concerning quality of life
4. Encouragement of postgraduate degrees in areas related to quality of life
5. Reporting of quality of life studies in the pharmaceutical press. (44)

There are numerous opportunities for pharmaceutical marketers to work with professional organizations; academe; providers of continuing education, residency, fellowship, and graduate programs; and the various pharmacy-related journals to provide education and information to the pharmacist concerning quality of life. At this crucial juncture in the development of HRQOL measurement in pharmacy, initiatives on the part of pharmaceutical marketers can lead to a pivotal role in what we believe to be the next phase in pharmacy practice. Pharmaceutical marketers have an extraordinary opportunity for a win-win-win situation for the pharmacy practitioner, the pharmaceutical marketer, and most importantly, the patient. First, however, pharmaceutical marketers must decide whether the potential role of the pharmacist in quality of life assessment should be perceived as a threat to be worked against or as a tremendous opportunity to work with the pharmacy community.

REFERENCES

1. Kotler P. Marketing management. 7th ed. Englewood Cliffs, NJ: Prentice-Hall, 1991.

2. Wheelen TL, Hunger JD. Strategic management and business policy. 5th ed. Reading, MA: Addison-Wesley Publishing, 1995.

3. Wilson IB, Cleary PD. Linking clinical variables with health-related quality of life: a conceptual model of patient outcomes. JAMA 1995;273:59-65.

4. Wilson IB, Kaplan S. Clinical practice and patients' health status: how are the two related? Med Care 1995;33:AS209-14.

5. Kozma CM, Reeder CE, Schulz RM. Economic, clinical, and humanistic outcomes: a planning model for pharmacoeconomic research. Clin Ther 1993;15:1121-32.

6. Kozma CM. Outcomes research and pharmacy practice. Am Pharm 1995; NS35(7):35-41.

7. Sloan FA, Khakoo R, Cluff LE, Waldman RH. The impact of infectious and allergic diseases on the quality of life. Soc Sci Med 1979;13:473-82.

8. Jonsson B. Assessment of quality of life in chronic diseases. Acta Paediatr Scand Suppl 1987;337:164-9.

9. Ellwood PM. Shattuck lecture—outcomes management. A technology of patient experience. N Engl J Med 1988;318:1549-56.

10. Kazis LE. Health outcome assessments in medicine: history, applications, and new directions. Adv Intern Med 1991;36:109-30.

11. Bergner M. Measurement of health status. Med Care 1985;23:696-704.

12. Smart CR, Yates JW. Quality of life. Cancer 1987;60:620-2.

13. Lohr KN. Outcome measurement: concepts and questions. Inquiry 1988;25:37-50.

14. Revicki DA. Health-related quality of life in the evaluation of medical therapy for chronic illness. J Fam Pract 1989;29:377-80.

15. Revicki DA. Quality of life research and the health care industry. J Res Pharm Econ 1990;2(1):41-53.

16. Cheatle MD. The effect of chronic orthopedic infection on quality of life. Orthop Clin North Am 1991;22:539-47.

17. Yergan J, LoGerfo J, Shortell S, et al. Health status as a measure of need for medical care: a critique. Med Care 1981;19:57-68.

18. Najman JM, Levine S. Evaluating the impact of medical care and technologies on the quality of life: a review and critique. Soc Sci Med [F] 1981;15:107-15.

19. Drummond MF. Resource allocation decisions in health care: a role for quality of life assessments? J Chron Dis 1987;40:605-19.

20. Bloom JR. Quality of life after cancer. A policy perspective. Cancer 1991;67:855-9.

21. Lohr KN. Applications of health status assessment measures in clinical practice. Overview of the third conference on advances in health status assessment. Med Care 1992;30:MS1-14.

22. Thier SO. Forces motivating the use of health status assessment measures in clinical settings and related clinical research. Med Care 1992;30:MS15-22.

23. Greenfield S, Nelson EC. Recent developments and future issues in the use of health status assessment measures in clinical settings. Med Care 1992;30:MS23-41.

24. Spiegelhalter DJ, Gore SM, Fitzpatrick R, et al. Quality of life measures in health care. III: resource allocation. Br Med J 1992;305:1205-9.

25. Donovan JL, Frankel SJ, Eyles JD. Assessing the need for health status measures. J Epidemiol Community Health 1993;47:158-62.

26. Guyatt GH, Feeny DH, Patrick DL. Measuring health-related quality of life. Ann Intern Med 1993;118:622-9.

27. Nelson E, Conger B, Douglass R, et al. Functional health status levels of primary care patients. JAMA 1983;249:3331-8.

28. Calkins DR, Rubenstein LV, Cleary PD, et al. Failure of physicians to recognize functional disability in ambulatory patients. Ann Intern Med 1991;114:451-4.

29. Sprangers MAG, Aaronson NK. The role of health care providers and significant others in evaluating the quality of life of patients with chronic disease: a review. J Clin Epidemiol 1992;45:743-60.

30. American Pharmaceutical Association. The mission of pharmacy. Pharmacy Update 1991;April 29:5+.

31. Hepler CD, Strand LM. Opportunities and responsibilities in pharmaceutical care. Am J Hosp Pharm 1990;47:533-43.

32. Reeder CE. Economic outcomes and contemporary pharmacy practice. Am Pharm 1993;NS33(12 Suppl):S3-6.

33. Osterhaus RJ, Osterhaus MC. Community pharmacy and health care research. Am Pharm 1991;NS31(3):40-1.

34. American Society of Hospital Pharmacists. ASHP Statement on Pharmaceutical Care. Practice Standards of ASHP, 1993-1994. Bethesda, MD: American Society of Hospital Pharmacists, 1995.

35. Smith M, Juergens J, Jack W. Medication and the quality of life. Am Pharm 1991;NS31(4):27-33.

36. Bentley JP. A study of the feasibility of the utilization of health-related quality of life instruments in the community pharmacy setting [Thesis]. University, MS: University of Mississippi, 1996.

37. Bergner M, Barry MJ, Bowman MA, et al. Where do we go from here? Opportunities for applying health status assessment measures in clinical settings. Med Care 1992;30:MS219-30.

38. Knapp DA. Barriers faced by pharmacists when attempting to maximize their contribution to society. Am J Pharm Educ 1979;43:357-9.

39. Kusserow RP. The clinical role of the community pharmacist. OAI-01-89-89160. Washington, DC: Office of the Inspector General, 1990.

40. Penna RP. Pharmaceutical care: pharmacy's mission for the 1990s. Am J Hosp Pharm 1990;47:543-9.

41. Raisch DW. Barriers to providing cognitive services. Am Pharm 1993; NS33(12):54-8.

42. Miller MJ, Ortmeier BG. Factors influencing the delivery of pharmacy services. Am Pharm 1995;NS35(1):39-45.

43. Jack W. Pharmaceutical differentiation through quality of life measurement: a case study. J Pharm Market Manage 1991;6(1):65-85.

44. Salek MS. Health-related quality of life measurement: a new challenge for pharmacy practitioners. J Pharm Pharmacol 1993;45:387-92.

45. Angaran DM. Quality assurance to quality improvement: measuring and monitoring pharmaceutical care. Am J Hosp Pharm 1991;48:1901-7.

46. Hayry M. Measuring the quality of life: why, how and what? Theor Med 1991; 12:97-116.

47. Jaeschke R, Guyatt GH, Cook D. Quality of life instruments in the evaluation of new drugs. PharmacoEconomics 1992;1:84-94.

48. Martin DP, Gilson BS, Bergner M, et al. The sickness impact profile: potential use of a health status instrument for physician training. J Med Educ 1976;51:942-4.

49. Ware JE, Brook RH, Davies AR, Lohr KN. Choosing measures of health status for individuals in general populations. Am J Public Health 1981;71:620-5.

50. Levine S. The changing terrains in medical sociology: emergent concern with quality of life. J Health Soc Behav 1987;28:1-6.

51. Rubenstein LV, Calkins DR, Greenfield S, et al. Health status assessment for elderly patients. Report of the Society of General Internal Medicine Task Force on Health Assessment. J Am Geriatr Soc 1989;37:562-9.

52. Patrick DL, Bergner M. Measurement of health status in the 1990s. Annu Rev Public Health 1990;11:165-83.

53. Fitzpatrick R, Fletcher A, Gore S, et al. Quality of life measures in health care. I: applications and issues in assessment. Br Med J 1992;305:1074-7.

54. Kirshner B, Guyatt G. A methodological framework for assessing health indices. J Chron Dis 1985;38:27-36.

55. Ware JE. Measures for a new era of health assessment. In: Stewart AL, Ware JE, eds. Measuring functioning and well-being: the medical outcomes approach. Durham, NC: Duke University Press, 1992:3-11.

56. Nelson E, Wasson J, Kirk J et al. Assessment of function in routine clinical practice: description of the COOP chart method and preliminary findings. J Chron Dis 1987;40:55S-63S.

57. Applegate WB. Use of assessment instruments in clinical settings. J Am Geriatr Soc 1987;35:45-50.

58. Nelson EC, Berwick DM. The measurement of health status in clinical practice. Med Care 1989;27:S77-89.

59. Nelson EC, Landgraf JM, Hays RD, et al. The functional status of patients: how can it be measured in physicians' offices. Med Care 1990;28:1111-23.

60. Keith RA. Functional status and health status. Arch Phys Med Rehabil 1994; 75:478-83.

61. Meyer KB, Espindle DM, DeGiacomo JM, et al. Monitoring dialysis patients' health status. Am J Kidney Dis 1994;24:267-79.

62. McHorney CA, Tarlov AR. Individual-patient monitoring in clinical practice: are available health status surveys adequate? Qual Life Res 1995;4:293-307.

63. Ganz PA. Impact of quality of life outcomes on clinical practice. Oncology (Huntingt) 1995;9(11 Suppl):61-5.

64. Wagner AK, Vickrey BG. The routine use of health-related quality of life measures in the care of patients with epilepsy: rationale and research agenda. Qual Life Res 1995;4:169-77.

65. Terry K. Can functional-status surveys improve your care? Med Econ 1996; 73(15):126+.

66. Deyo RA, Carter WB. Strategies for improving and expanding the application of health status measures in clinical settings. Med Care 1992;30:MS176-86.

67. Calkins DR, Rubenstein LV, Cleary PD, et al. The Functional Status Questionnaire: a controlled trial in a hospital-based practice. Clin Res 1986;34:359A.

68. Rubenstein LV, Calkins DR, Young RT, et al. Improving patient functional status: can questionnaires help? Clin Res 1986;34:835A.

69. Rubenstein LV, Calkins DR, Young RT, et al. Improving patient function: a randomized trial of functional disability screening. Ann Intern Med 1989;111: 836-42.

70. Kazis LE, Callahan LF, Meenan RF, Pincus T. Health status reports in the care of patients with rheumatoid arthritis. J Clin Epidemiol 1990;43:1243-53.

71. Rubenstein LV, McCoy JM, Cope DW, et al. Improving patient quality of life with feedback to physicians about functional status. J Gen Intern Med 1995;10: 607-14.

72. Rubenstein L. The clinical effectiveness of multidimensional geriatric assessment. J Am Geriatr Soc 1983;31:758-62.

73. American College of Physicians. Comprehensive functional assessment for elderly patients. Ann Intern Med 1988;110:70-2.

74. MacKeigan LD, Pathak DS. Overview of health-related quality of life measures. Am J Hosp Pharm 1992;49:2236-45.

75. McCorvey EJ, Wright JTJ, Culbert JP, et al. Effect of hydrochlorothiazide, enalapril, and propranolol on quality of life and cognitive and motor function in hypertensive patients. Clin Pharm 1993;12:300-5.

76. Fowlie M, Berkeley J. Quality of life–a review of the literature. Fam Pract 1987;4:226-34.

77. Goodinson SM, Singleton J. Quality of life: a critical review of current concepts, measures and their clinical implications. Int J Nurs Stud 1989;26:327-41.

78. McCauley C, Bremer BA. Subjective quality of life measures for evaluating medical intervention. Eval Health Prof 1991;14:371-87.

79. Meenan RF. The AIMS approach to health status measurement: conceptual background and measurement properties. J Rheumatol 1982;9:785-8.

80. LeMay P. Quality of life–measuring outcomes of pharmaceutical management. Summary of workshop proceedings. Can J Public Health 1992;83:S5-16.

81. Coons SJ, Kaplan RM. Assessing health-related quality of life: application to drug therapy. Clin Ther 1992;14:850-8.

82. Bergner M, Bobbitt RA, Carter WB, Gilson BS. The Sickness Impact Profile: development and final revision of a health status measure. Med Care 1981;19: 787-805.

83. Guyatt GH, Veldhuyzen Van Zanten SJO, Feeny DH, Patrick DL. Measuring quality of life in clinical trials: a taxonomy and review. Can Med Assoc J 1989;140: 1441-8.

84. Pathak DS, MacKeigan LD. Assessment of quality of life and health status: selected observations. J Res Pharm Econ 1992;4(4):31-52.

85. Wilkin D, Hallam L, Doggett M. Measures of need and outcome for primary health care. New York: Oxford University Press, 1992.

86. Bungay KM, Ware JE. Measuring and monitoring health-related quality of life. Kalamazoo, MI: The Upjohn Company, 1993.

87. Hays RD, Anderson R, Revicki D. Psychometric considerations in evaluating health-related quality of life measures. Qual Life Res 1993;2:441-9.

88. Streiner DL, Norman GR. Health measurement scales: a practical guide to their development and use. 2nd ed. New York: Oxford University Press, 1995.

89. McDowell I, Newell C. Measuring health: a guide to rating scales and questionnaires. 2nd ed. New York: Oxford University Press, 1996.

90. Spilker B, ed. Quality of life and pharmacoeconomics in clinical trials. 2nd ed. Philadelphia, PA: Lippincott-Raven Publishers, 1996.

91. Bungay KM, Wagner AK. Comment: assessing the quality of pharmaceutical care. Ann Pharmacother 1993;27:1542.

92. Jette AM, Davies AR, Cleary PD, et al. The Functional Status Questionnaire: reliability and validity when used in primary care. J Gen Intern Med 1986;1:143-9.

93. Hunt SM, McKenna SP, McEwen J, et al. A quantitative approach to perceived health status: a validation study. J Epidemiol Community Health 1980;34: 281-6.

94. Parkerson GR, Broadhead WE, Tse CK. The Duke Health Profile: a 17-item measure of health and dysfunction. Med Care 1990;28:1056-72.

95. Ware JE, Sherbourne CD. The MOS 36-item short-form health survey (SF-36) I. Conceptual framework and item selection. Med Care 1992;30:473-81.

96. McHorney CA, Ware JE, Raczek AE. The MOS 36-item short-form health survey (SF-36) II. Psychometric and clinical tests of validity in measuring physical and mental health constructs. Med Care 1993;31:247-63.

97. McHorney CA, Ware JE, Lu JFR, et al. The MOS 36-item short-form health survey (SF-36) III. Tests of data quality, scaling assumptions, and reliability across diverse patient groups. Med Care 1994;32:40-66.

98. Rector TS. Patients' assessment of outcomes: an important aspect of pharmaceutical care. J Pharm Teach 1992;3(3):21-7.

99. Devinsky O. Clinical uses of the quality-of-life in epilepsy inventory. Epilepsia 1993;34(Suppl 4):S39-44.

100. Cramer JA. Quality of life for people with epilepsy. Neurol Clin 1994;12: 1-13.

101. Ware J, Kosinski M, Keller SD. A 12-item short-form health survey: construction of scales and preliminary tests of reliability and validity. Med Care 1996;34: 220-33.

102. Health Status Questionnaire (HSQ) 2.0 user guide. Bloomington, MN: Health Outcomes Institute, 1993.

103. Segal ME, Schall RR. Determining functional/health status and its relation to disability in stroke survivors. Stroke 1994;25:2391-7.

104. Nunnally J. Psychometric theory. 2nd ed. New York: McGraw-Hill, 1978.

105. Prisant LM, Carr AA, Bottini PB, et al. Repeatability of automated ambulatory blood pressure measurements. J Fam Pract 1992;34:569-74.

106. Lindley CM, Hirsch JD. Oncology nurses' attitudes, perceptions, and knowledge of quality-of-life assessment in patients with cancer. Oncol Nurs Forum 1994; 21:103-8.

Trends in Patient Counseling and Education

John P. Juergens

BACKGROUND

The provision of useful drug information to patients, verbally or written, concerns the Food and Drug Administration (FDA), health care professionals, pharmaceutical manufacturers, managed care organizations, and consumers. This is not a particularly new trend for pharmacists, since advising patients on proper medication use has always been a primary function of the profession. However, as the popularity of self-medication, consumerism, and direct-to-consumer advertising (DTCA) has increased, the quality, availability, and usefulness of patient counseling efforts and information sources have become key considerations to a much broader audience.

Although providing patients with advice about their medications is a pillar of the profession, the FDA has long been concerned that patients were not consistently receiving adequate information from pharmacists, physicians, and nurses about their increasingly potent prescription medications and that this lack of patient education was contributing to unnecessary and avoidable morbidity and mortality for patients as well as increasing the burden of health care costs (1). For many years, the agency also believed that some prescription medications warranted additional written information to enhance patient

John P. Juergens, Ph.D., is Research Associate Professor, Research Institute of Pharmaceutical Sciences, and Associate Professor of Pharmacy Administration, School of Pharmacy, University of Mississippi, University, MS 38677.

[Haworth co-indexing entry note]: "Trends in Patient Counseling and Education." Juergens, John P. Co-published simultaneously in *Journal of Pharmaceutical Marketing Practice* (Pharmaceutical Products Press, an imprint of The Haworth Press, Inc.) Vol. 1, No. 2 (#2), 1998, pp. 117-129; and: *Marketing to Pharmacists: Understanding Their Role and Influence* (ed: Benjamin F. Banahan III) Pharmaceutical Products Press, an imprint of The Haworth Press, Inc., 1998, pp. 117-129. Single or multiple copies of this article are available for a fee from The Haworth Document Delivery Service [1-800-342-9678, 9:00 a.m. - 5:00 p.m. (EST). E-mail address: getinfo@haworthpressinc.com].

education on the proper use of those drugs. Since 1968, printed patient information leaflets, or PPIs, have been mandated for several types of drugs, including oral contraceptives, estrogens, and inhaled isoproterenol (2). At one point the FDA also considered requiring printed information for a wide variety of other prescription drugs; however, after evaluating the opinions of health care professionals, the FDA abandoned this idea. Issues concerning storage, pharmacist liability, and the lack of documentation of benefit to patients (i.e., no increase in compliance or improvement in health care outcome) were the primary arguments cited by pharmacists against mandatory medication guides for all prescriptions (3). The agency also concluded that mandatory requirements were unnecessary because the goal of improved patient education could be achieved through private-sector initiatives.

In the decade following the withdrawal of the PPI regulations, the FDA maintained its vigilance on this issue and conducted research to evaluate the progress made by the voluntary private-sector programs on the development of patient medication educational materials. The results of that research showed minimal progress in improving the distribution of printed prescription drug information (4). Consequently, the FDA made the provision of patient information a key goal in the 1990's by promoting the distribution of patient information leaflets with prescriptions and the development of innovative drug information software by pharmacy chain organizations to complement verbal counseling (5).

RECENT TRENDS

Concern for patient education was codified in 1990 with the passage of the Omnibus Budget Reconciliation Act (OBRA '90), which contained a provision mandating oral patient counseling for Medicaid patients about their prescription medications. Since the passage of that bill, ensuring the availability of accurate and understandable drug, disease, and health information for all patients has become an important goal for all parties involved in the delivery of health care. The results of consumer surveys conducted by the FDA to determine the extent to which patients receive written medication information from pharmacists along with verbal counseling is shown in Figure 1. A dramatic upward trend in the percentage of consumers reporting receiving medication information occurred after the 1993 implementation of the OBRA '90 counseling requirements.

FIGURE 1. Receipt of Written Information at the Pharmacy.

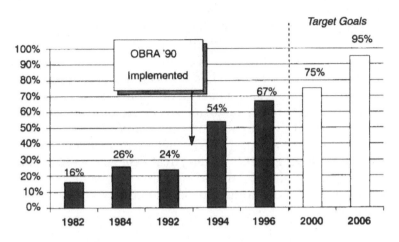

Source: FDA, National Consumer Surveys, 1982-1996. As developed by the National Council on Patient Information and Education, Washington, DC: *The NCPIE News* (Spring, 1997). Reprinted with the permission.

Similar surveys were conducted by other organizations that attempted to assess the utility of the information provided (6). In a 1994 survey, the National Association of Boards of Pharmacy (NABP) found that 64% of consumers reported receiving written information, and the majority (92%) of those individuals said that they had read the information and that it was clear and easy to understand. In a 1996 survey, the American Pharmaceutical Association (APhA) found that 81% of consumers surveyed reported always receiving written information with their new prescription medication. Of those receiving information, 69% indicated that they read all or most of the information, and of these respondents 75% said the information was "very useful."

Acknowledging that good progress had been achieved in some areas of patient education, the FDA, seeking to bolster its commitment to patient medication education, in 1995 published a proposed rule, the "MedGuide Requirements," which aimed to increase uniformly the quality and quantity of written information about prescription medications (1). The FDA's proposal would have required manufacturers to produce MedGuides for certain medications that pose a serious and significant public health concern. The proposal also encouraged written information leaflets to be produced for all drugs and distributed by physicians and pharmacists. Goals were established that useful information should reach 75% of individuals receiving new prescriptions by the year 2000 and 95% of individuals by the year 2006.

Subsequent to this direct intervention by the FDA in the patient information and education issue, it has been recognized that not only can the level of general health and quality of life increase for patients, but there also is a potential to reduce therapeutic noncompliance, adverse drug events, hospitalization, and health care usage costs with enhanced patient education (1). The notion of reducing health care costs while improving quality of care, treatment outcomes, and quality of life has inherent practical marketing value with significant implications for pharmacists, pharmaceutical manufacturers, and marketing organizations.

ECONOMIC ASPECTS OF PPIs

The benefits of education programs for patients are intuitively positive and have been documented in several research studies (6-10). One of the most comprehensive studies, conducted by the Rand Corporation, showed that patients read and used drug information as a reference and that the information reliably increased patients' knowledge and understanding of their drugs (4). However, it has also been demonstrated that increasing patient drug knowledge does not necessarily translate into therapeutic compliance and improved outcomes as measured by biological parameters (11, 12).

Reid has stated that there is a difference between drug information and drug education (13). Drug information provides factual data about drugs and diseases, while drug education implies understanding and integrating drug therapy into a behavioral change. Reid also suggested that a combination of information and education is necessary for effective patient counseling. For example, Etzwiler and Robb evaluated an educational program for juvenile diabetics and their families (14). After the intervention, the researchers found a significant increase in knowledge of the disease and techniques for self-management but found no improvement in the control of the disease as measured by blood and urine glucose levels. The authors concluded that, "It would be naive to assume or suggest that an accumulation of facts by consumers will ensure proper control of any disease process." They also suggested that, once educated, patients must be motivated and supported to carry out proper medical management of their diseases.

The need for motivation and follow-up support is reinforced by the work of Merritt et al., who demonstrated that comprehensive patient education programs, when integrated into patient therapeutic management, can improve patients' health as measured by biological parameters (15). In this study, the researchers developed a clinic for diabetic patients and their families that provided comprehensive education about the disease along with recurring support and motivation from the clinic staff, which included a physician, clinical pharmacist, clinical dietician, diabetes teaching nurse, and podiatrist. The program emphasized patients' responsibility in controlling their disease and, ultimately, its impact on their quality of life. Long-term assessment of the educational support program demonstrated a 23% reduction in the rate of hospital admissions among the study population for uncontrolled diabetes.

The economic value of a multifaceted educational approach to enhance long-term compliance was demonstrated by Sclar et al. (16). This study was designed to determine the effect of health education on the utilization of health services for hypertension. HMO patients with existing hypertension and those newly diagnosed with mild to moderate hypertension who met certain inclusion criteria were enrolled in a program consisting of an educational newsletter, information about nutrition and lifestyle change, verbal counseling, and motivational reinforcement. In addition to this educational component, the program also included a 30-day supply of medication, refill reminder postcards, and samples and coupons for health-related items.

Statistical analysis of the impact of the various program components indicated that the educational program was associated with a decrease in aggregate health care costs of $127.79 during the study period for patients with existing hypertension and $92.97 for newly diagnosed patients as compared to patients in the control group. In both cases, these savings were the result of an increase in expenditures for prescription drugs and a decrease in the use of physician, laboratory, and hospital services.

Although intuition and some empirical research support the value of printed medication information, studies showing no effect on compliance or biological parameters raise questions about the costs of producing and distributing these materials relative to their benefits in terms of useful outcomes. If we cannot demonstrate that patient-oriented drug and disease information reliably contributes directly to improved therapeutic outcomes, can we justify the cost associated with using these materials?

As described above, several recent studies have been conducted to estimate the actual costs and financial benefits associated with patient counseling and comprehensive, multifaceted education strategies that include printed information materials. However, no recent studies have been identified that evaluate the economic costs and benefits associated specifically with printed education and counseling materials. On the basis of the literature currently available, it might not be possible–or desirable–to develop a single, general economic model for assessing the cost and benefits of the specific components of various patient education strategies. There may be a synergistic or reinforcing relationship among educational program components that prevents accurate quantification. This, along with the lack of standard methods of defining costs and benefits, may force us to conduct cost-benefit analyses on a case-by-case basis for individual patient education efforts.

USEFULNESS OF PPIs

As a result of the FDA's proposed MedGuide regulations and as progress has been made in the development of PPIs, there has been considerable interest in evaluating the utility of existing patient information, and research has been conducted to determine how to improve materials to meet FDA standards of "useful." ["Useful" is defined as enabling the patient to use the medication properly and appropriately, receive the maximum benefit from it, and avoid harm (5).]

Printed medication materials are available from a wide range of sources, including pharmaceutical manufacturers, consumer groups and associations, and commercial information vendors. Although all of the providers of printed medication information have the same basic goal of supplying consumers with more and better information about their prescription medications, each operates under somewhat different constraints. These constraints have an effect on the presentation and content of the materials the providers produce. For example, information leaflets supplied by manufacturers must meet stringent review criteria established by the FDA, since those documents are considered part of the product labeling. Hence, the kinds of information and the manner in which it is presented in such PPIs can differ substantially from the information and presentation developed by commercial information vendors who are not covered by FDA regulations. Furthermore, there is no consensus among the FDA, the pharmaceutical industry, the medical and pharmacy communities, and consumer groups on the appropriate content of printed patient medication information. Consequently, there is a lack of consistency in the quality and utility of available patient education materials.

In 1993, Basara and Juergens conducted a study to assess consumers' desire for medication information, to determine the proportion of those receiving information from their pharmacist, and to characterize the currently available patient information leaflets in terms of readability and "user friendliness" (17). When asked about their desire to receive information about their medications and illness, 90% of all respondents wanted to know as much as possible about their drug therapy. On the other hand, just over half (52%) of the respondents indicated that they received such information from their pharmacist.

Readability was evaluated for PPIs from three sources: pharmaceutical manufacturers of brand-name products, nonprofit health care organizations, and commercial sources of patient information. The results indicated substantial variability in the accessibility of the information contained in the study sample of patient medication leaflets and suggested that most of the printed information available at that time needed improvement. As indicated in Table 1, the average PPI reading level (9th grade) was substantially higher than the recommended reading level for consumer materials, which is 6th to 8th grade. PPIs of commercial vendors generally were the most difficult to read if evaluated according to grade level and reading ease analysis, while pharmaceutical company PPIs were slightly less difficult. Association PPIs were the easiest to read, with an average reading level at about the 7th grade.

User friendliness of PPIs was assessed qualitatively and quantitatively by means of an index composed of values for the PPI features of print size, use of graphics and color printing, amount of white space, and paper quality. Overall, it was found that most PPIs evaluated did not contain graphics, were printed in one color of ink, and had small type or poor print quality (Table 2). Although few PPIs included

TABLE 1. Results of PPI Readability Analysis.

PPI Source	Mean Reading Level	
	FRE*	FK**
Pharmaceutical companies	58.4	9.1
Vendors	52.7	9.0
Associations	62.5	7.4
Total	**56.6**	**8.8**

*Flesch Reading Ease (FRE) measures readability on a 100-point scale. As the score decreases, readability increases. Scores in the 50-60 range are estimated to require a ninth to tenth grade reading level.

**Flesch-Kincaid (FK) measures readability using the same methods as the FRE, but translates the results to grade level for easier interpretation.

Reprinted with permission from Basara LR, Juergens JP. Patient package insert readability and design. Am Pharm 1994; NS34(8):48-53.

TABLE 2. User-Friendliness Index Results by PPI Source.

Source	UFI	
	Average	Range
Pharmaceutical companies	7.16	5-12
Vendors	7.59	7-13
Associations	8.9	8-11

Scale: 5 to 13, where 5 = poorly designed and 13 = optimally designed

Reprinted with permission from Basara LR, Juergens JP. Patient package insert readability and design. Am Pharm 1994; NS34(8):48-53.

graphics, those produced by commercial vendors used the most. Most PPIs from pharmaceutical companies and associations did not include graphics, even though graphics are important for emphasizing instructions and illustrating administration techniques, such as how to use inhalers or transdermal patches.

In 1994, Juergens and Basara conducted a second study that consisted of a national survey of community pharmacists to determine quantitatively community pharmacists' perceptions of the relative utility of current printed patient information; to obtain pharmacists' perspectives on the appropriate content of patient medication guides; and to determine community pharmacists' preferences for future patient information materials in terms of content, format, source, and adaptability (18).

In general, pharmacists believed their patients wanted printed information that would help inform them about their medications and diseases. However, there was strong evidence that current materials are not sufficient for present and future counseling needs. Understandability of printed patient information was a primary concern for pharmacists, and they believed materials need to be adaptable to suit individual patient needs. Many pharmacists believed that patient literacy level is a serious barrier to effective patient counseling and estimated that less than one-fourth of their patients read and understand the medication information provided to them. While pharmacists did not want patient information materials regulated by the FDA, they preferred consistent materials in terms of standardized formats, content, etc. Despite their concerns, it was encouraging that the large majority of pharmacists have a very positive attitude toward patient counseling as indicated in the survey.

The overall goals of patient education and counseling are to promote safe and effective use of all types of medical and medication therapy, promote medication compliance, reduce symptoms, improve therapeutic outcomes and health, and ultimately improve patients' perceived and actual quality of life. All of these goals have inherent implications for patients, health professionals, health care organizations, pharmaceutical manufacturers, marketing agencies, and society in general. The goals of patient education are consistent with the national interest and the desire to control health care costs while maintaining or improving quality of care and quality of life.

EMERGING TRENDS AND OPPORTUNITIES

On August 6, 1996, Public Law 104-180 was passed, which required the Secretary of Health and Human Services to organize a committee of diverse interests to develop a long-range, comprehensive action plan to improve oral and written communications to patients about their prescription medications. A steering committee was formed, and an action plan was developed and submitted to the Secretary of HHS in December 1996 and accepted in January 1997. This action plan set forth a detailed process by which the private sector would work to improve the quality and availability of useful information that is voluntarily provided to consumers with their prescription medication. Acceptance of this action plan by the Secretary had the effect of rescinding the FDA's authority to implement the proposed MedGuide regulations described above. As required by P.L. 104-180, the action plan addresses the following issues:

1. Assess the effectiveness of the current private-sector approaches used to provide oral and written prescription information to consumers
2. Develop guidelines for providing effective oral and written prescription information consistent with the findings of any such assessment
3. Contain elements necessary to ensure the transmittal of useful information to the consuming public, including being scientifically accurate, nonpromotional in tone and content, sufficiently specific and comprehensive as to adequately inform consumers about the use of the product, and in an understandable, legible format that is readily comprehensible and not confusing to consumers expected to use the product
4. Develop a mechanism to assess periodically the quality of the oral and written prescription information and the frequency with which the information is provided to consumers
5. Provide for compliance with relevant state board regulations. (5)

While the private sector has taken upon itself the responsibility of maximizing the potential of patient education and counseling, it is clear that the pharmacist is a key component in realizing that potential. In their expanding role as patient therapeutic counselors, pharmacists require targeted, consistent, and effective tools to ensure patients receive the medication information they need and desire in a functional format. Just as a carpenter cannot build a cabinet with improper tools, a community pharmacist cannot counsel patients with inappropriate or ineffectual materials. If pharmacists are aware of the design considerations that affect the utility of printed medication information and the potential for misinterpretation of that information, they will be in a position to select, develop, and present counseling materials in the most effective manner for a given patient. PPIs also present an opportunity for community pharmacists to enhance their professional image and to differentiate their service by distributing high-quality, high-utility patient information materials with the prescription medications they dispense. Although the results of several studies suggest that progress is being made in patient counseling and education, pharmacists currently do not appear to have the best tools to counsel their patients effectively on the broad range of needs presented. In addition, pharmacists are concerned that current patient information materials will not be adequate for future counseling needs. Therefore, it is important for pharmacists to communicate these issues to pharmaceutical manufacturers, software vendors, and other organizations that produce patient-oriented medication information and counseling materials.

Many pharmaceutical manufacturers, software vendors, and other organizations produce patient-oriented medication information. Improvements are needed in readability, which can be quantitatively measured, and in understandability, which requires a more qualitative assessment by the end user of the materials. This suggests that there are product differentiation opportunities for producers of PPIs. Because counseling requirements have increased the demands on pharmacists' time, anything manufacturers or suppliers of patient information materials can do to facilitate the counseling process will be well-received. Pharmacists, the primary conduit through which patient education materials flow, are more likely to use products that are accompanied by a complete patient counseling support package that makes more efficient use of their time.

For managed care organizations, there appears to be sufficient documented evidence of the potential economic benefits of PPIs to warrant their use in comprehensive patient education and disease and therapy management programs. Several studies have demonstrated substantial reductions in the utilization of expensive health care services, as well as genuine improvement in the course of disease. Widespread use of multifaceted education programs could be an effective strategy in reducing overall health care costs.

The pharmaceutical industry faces some enormous challenges in the endorsed action plan for patient education. We must keep in mind that even if patients are able to read the words, if they do not understand what is being presented, then, at best, they remain uneducated, and, at worst, they are confused or frightened into deeper noncompliance. It appears that the FDA plans to allow the industry some latitude in producing patient education materials with respect to labeling regulations. With fewer hurdles, manufacturers can produce materials that are appropriate, useful, and understandable, rather than producing legal documents.

Finally, while the benefits of verbal counseling of patients are well-known, continued research is needed to assess and document the impact of printed medical information on compliance, health outcomes, and medical cost reduction and the costs of producing and distributing PPIs. However, we must recognize the possibility that, within the context of the action plan mandates, continued research could demonstrate that PPIs improve therapeutic outcomes but at costs that exceed savings. Barring this finding, the significant increase in product-related expenses that patient medication information represents for pharmaceutical manufacturers will be better justified in light of data that demonstrate a favorable cost-benefit ratio associated with their use as part of a comprehensive educational effort.

REFERENCES

1. Prescription drug product labeling: medication guide requirements. Fed Reg 1995;60(164):44182.

2. Morris L. Patient package inserts: a new tool for patient education. Public Health Rep 1977;92:421-4.

3. Johnson M, Mitch W, Sherwood J, et al. The impact of a drug information sheet on the understandability and attitude of patients about drugs. JAMA 1986;256: 2722-4.

4. Drug industry efforts to communicate with patients should focus on education after prescription is dispensed, FDA Commissioner tells NACDS. FDC Rep–Pink Sheet 1992;(Sept 7):9-10.

5. Steering Committee for the Collaborative Development of a Long-Rang Action Plan for the Provision of Useful Prescription Medicine Information. Action plan for the provision of useful prescription medicine information. Keystone, CO: The Keystone Center, December, 1996.

6. Joubert P, Lasagna L. Patient package inserts: nature, notions, and needs. Clin Pharm Ther 1975;18:507-13.

7. Fleckenstein L. Attitudes toward the patient package insert–a survey of physicians and pharmacists. Drug Info J 1977;11:23-9.

8. Morris L. Rationale for patient package inserts. Am J Hosp Pharm 1978;35: 179-84.

9. Mazis M, Morris L, Gordon E. Patient attitudes about two forms of printed oral contraceptive information. Med Care 1978;16:1045-54.

10. Weintraub M, Glickstein S, Lasagna L. Estrogen patient package insert: medication acceptance despite negative attitudes. Clin Pharm Ther 1981;30:149-53.

11. Webb P. Effectiveness of patient education and psychosocial counseling in promoting compliance and control among hypertensive patients. J Fam Pract 1980; 10:1047-55.

12. Zahr L, Yazigi A, Armenian H. The effect of education and written material on compliance of pediatric clients. Intern J Nurs Stud 1989;26:213-20.

13. Reid L. Here are 4 basic ways to improve patient compliance. Wellcome Trends in Pharmacy 1992;14(Sept):5.

14. Etzweiler D, Robb J. Evaluation of programmed education among juvenile diabetics and their families. Diabetes 1972;21:967-71.

15. Merrit G, Kobernus C, Hall N, et al. Outcomes analysis of a diabetic education clinic. Mil Med 1983;148:545-7.

16. Sclar D, Skaer T, Chin A, et al. Effect of health education on the utilization of HMO services: a prospective trial among patients with hypertension. Prim Card 1992;18(Suppl 1):3034.

17. Basara L, Juergens J. Patient package insert readability and design: research results and practice implications. Am Pharm 1994;NS34:48-53.

18. Juergens J, Basara L. Patient information: community pharmacy needs and perspectives. Top Hosp Pharm 1994;14:47-57.

Current Perspectives: Establishing Relationships with Pharmacists

John P. Bentley
Benjamin F. Banahan III

INTRODUCTION

Few would argue that a primary function of marketing is "mobilizing an organization's resources to satisfy customer needs," and few would dispute the need to develop cooperative, long-term relationships with customers to gain competitive advantages in the marketplace (1). However, who are the customers of the pharmaceutical industry? In other words, whose needs should pharmaceutical marketers attempt to satisfy and with whom should pharmaceutical marketers establish relationships?

Historically, the customer of the pharmaceutical industry was the physician, as it was the physician who created product demand and

John P. Bentley, M.B.A., M.S., is Graduate Research Assistant, Research Institute of Pharmaceutical Sciences, and a graduate student in the Department of Pharmacy Administration, School of Pharmacy, University of Mississippi, University, MS 38677. E-mail: phjpb@olemiss.edu.

Benjamin F. Banahan III, Ph.D., is Research Professor and Coordinator for the Pharmaceutical Marketing and Management Research Program, Research Institute of Pharmaceutical Sciences, and Professor of Pharmacy Administration, School of Pharmacy, University of Mississippi.

[Haworth co-indexing entry note]: "Current Perspectives: Establishing Relationships with Pharmacists." Bentley, John P., and Benjamin F. Banahan III. Co-published simultaneously in *Journal of Pharmaceutical Marketing Practice* (Pharmaceutical Products Press, an imprint of The Haworth Press, Inc.) Vol. 1, No. 2 (#2), 1998, pp. 131-150; and: *Marketing to Pharmacists: Understanding Their Role and Influence* (ed: Benjamin F. Banahan III) Pharmaceutical Products Press, an imprint of The Haworth Press, Inc., 1998, pp. 131-150. Single or multiple copies of this article are available for a fee from The Haworth Document Delivery Service [1-800-342-9678, 9:00 a.m. - 5:00 p.m. (EST). E-mail address: getinfo@haworthpressinc.com].

131

who was the primary decision maker in the drug use process (2, 3). However, as the health care environment changed, so did the customer of the pharmaceutical industry. Pharmacists, managed care organizations, health care systems, regulators, and others have all grown in their importance as customers with respect to the pharmaceutical marketer. So, too, have patients. In fact, most would agree with John Gans, Executive Vice President of the American Pharmaceutical Association, who said that "the goal of all of us, whether it be the manufacturers, the regulators, the prescribers, or the dispensers, must be to assure that the patient who receives medication receives the maximum therapeutic outcome from its use. It is the patient–not the manufacturer, not the prescriber, not the pharmacist–who must be the ultimate beneficiary" (3). The question is, how can these diverse groups work together to achieve optimal patient outcomes? More specific to the purpose of this paper, how can pharmaceutical manufacturers and practitioners of pharmacy collaborate to improve the health of patients?

Although the pharmaceutical industry has its roots in pharmacy practice, the manufacturers of pharmaceuticals and pharmacy practitioners have traveled different paths (4). What was traditionally the art of pharmacy has been almost completely taken over by the pharmaceutical industry (5). In the 1930's, about 75% of prescriptions required some compounding by a pharmacist. By 1950, that figure had dropped to 25%, and by 1970, about 1 in 100 prescriptions required compounding by a pharmacist (6). Despite having their traditional function overtaken, pharmacists maintained a seemingly amicable relationship with manufacturers. These relationships were especially strong with some manufacturers, and the positive aspects were observed most frequently at the grassroots level, as individual pharmacists interacted with "local detailmen" (7, 8). Smith has observed that during the "Kefauver era there seemed to be a reasonably strong bond between the manufacturers and the retailers (perhaps because of a 'common enemy')" (8). However, over the past 30 years, a number of events have occurred that have not only strained the current relationship between pharmacists and manufacturers but have also made the possibility of establishing long-term, cooperative relationships more difficult.

The pharmacist's role in the health care system continues to evolve. No longer is the pharmacist simply the physician's "order taker." This evolution, in addition to other environmental changes, has led to the development of several conflicts between pharmacists and manufacturers. Despite the existence of conflicts between these groups, each has the opportunity to help the other achieve the overall goal of serving the patient. In addition to benefiting the ultimate consumer, both manufacturers and pharmacists have much to gain from establishing cooperative relationships.

The purpose of this last article in this issue is fivefold:

1. To demonstrate the value of establishing long-term, cooperative relationships with customers
2. To discuss past pharmaceutical marketing activities with respect to the pharmacist
3. To review the changes in the nature of the practice of pharmacy that have led several to conclude that more attention should be directed at establishing relationships with pharmacists
4. To offer suggestions of practices that pharmaceutical marketers can undertake to foster relationships with community pharmacists and to explore the potential benefits of such relationships
5. To examine methods by which pharmaceutical marketers can reach community pharmacists to establish relationships.

RELATIONSHIP MARKETING

Several authors have cited examples of conflicts that have occurred between the pharmacy community and pharmaceutical manufacturers over the past several years and have offered explanations for the apparent increase in strain in the relationship between these groups (9-12). The strain between these two pharmaceutical channel members is interesting in light of the fact that both marketing theory and marketing practice have undergone "a major directional change" in the past decade, turning toward the concept of relationship marketing and ushering in the relationship marketing era as a successor to the period in marketing defined by the marketing concept (13, 14). The general concept of managing relationships is not new to marketing or to the pharmaceutical industry; "[h]owever, the growing interest in relationship marketing suggests a shift in the nature of general marketplace transactions from discrete to relational exchanges–from exchanges between parties with no past history and no future to exchanges between parties who have an exchange history and plans for future interactions" (15).

Many have recognized that a requirement for being an effective competitor is that one must also be a trusted cooperator (13). Indeed, Weitz and Jap note that control mechanisms used to coordinate channel activities "are placing more emphasis on using relational norms and attitudes such as trust and commitment . . . rather than the use of authoritative control mechanisms or vertical integration" (15). Moreover, relationship marketing is characterized by the strategic perspective of putting the customer first: in essence, shifting the focus of marketing from manipulating the customer with telling and selling techniques to communicating and sharing knowledge with customers, establishing genuine customer involvement (16). The marketer no longer simply reacts to customer-initiated feedback but proactively initiates and maintains participative exchange with customers (14). As in the marketing of pharmaceuticals, the criteria for defining a customer have broadened. The customer is not only the end user of the product. Broadened definitions of relationship marketing call for establishing long-term relationships with any groups central to the success of the marketer (13).

The general benefits of engaging in relationship marketing become more apparent upon examination of its objectives: (1) the design of long-term relationships with customers to enhance value shares for both parties and (2) the extension of the long-term relationship idea to vertical and horizontal cooperation partners (17). Thus, value is created not only for the customer but for the marketer as well. In summary, relationship marketing calls for the establishment of close relationships that emphasize a long-term, win-win relationship based on mutual trust between customers and their suppliers (14).

A number of authors have focused on the establishment and maintenance of relationships and partnerships by various members of the pharmaceuticals distribution channel. For example, Doucette assesses potential opportunities for manufacturers and wholesalers, and Vitali encourages stronger relationships between these two channel members (18, 19). Harris and Scott describe partnerships between manufacturers and managed care organizations (20, 21). Although Joel notes that "[pharmaceutical] companies must create links with patients, physicians, *pharmacists*, and plan sponsors and effectively direct information to them to gain significant competitive advantage," (emphasis added) rarely is the pharmacist mentioned in the literature as a potential strategic partner for pharmaceutical manufacturers (22). While relationship marketing has typically referred to establishing close relationships with *individual* customers (treating each customer as a segment of one), it is not inconceivable to consider establishing relationships with larger segments, such as members of a profession (16). Indeed, relationship marketing in consumer markets, where it would be difficult for firms to establish close relationships with individual customers, has been explored (23-25).

The remainder of this paper explores the pharmacy profession, particularly those members who practice in a community setting, as a potential strategic partner for pharmaceutical manufacturers. Although the general emphasis is on forming relationships with the profession as a whole, this does not preclude the possibilities of establishing relationships with individual pharmacies or pharmacists. Before exploring practices that pharmaceutical marketers can undertake to foster relationships with this evolving market segment, it would be helpful to explore the historical relationship between manufacturers and pharmacists and how changes in the profession have altered this relationship.

PAST PHARMACEUTICAL MARKETING ACTIVITIES AND THE PHARMACIST

Historically, the pharmaceutical manufacturer distributed the product to the pharmacist but created demand through the physician by attempting to alter the prescribing process (2). The physician was the gatekeeper to pharmaceuticals and had a strong influence over the sale of the product through derived demand (2, 26). For these reasons, most marketing efforts were directed at the physician. Manufacturers spent a great deal of time and resources promoting products to physicians and expended a great deal of effort in trying to get to know and understand the physician. As Smith observed, "perhaps no other group in the United States or the world has been so thoroughly classified, categorized, and identified as has the American physician" (26).

This is not to say that information was not provided to the pharmacist by the manufacturer. However, the information provided to the pharmacist was usually of a commercial nature, whereas the information provided to the physician typically focused on clinical aspects such as safety and efficacy (2). The sales representative or "detailman" called on the pharmacist, but these calls were typically made to assure product availability or to inform the pharmacist about an upcoming pricing deal. Most companies had various service programs aimed at pharmacists, such as the *Lilly Digest* and the *Schering Reports*, usually operated by a pharmacy affairs department within the company (5). The manufacturer typically perceived the community pharmacist primarily as a retailer, however, rather than as a health care professional (26).

Relationships were developed between individual sales representatives and pharmacists, but these relationships typically revolved around the business aspects of the manufacturer and the pharmacy. Little attention was paid to the development of long-term, win-win relationships based on mutual trust; certainly the company (usually through the sales representative) reacted to customer-initiated feedback, but rarely did the company proactively initiate and maintain participative exchange with customers. The pharmacist was a channel member with minimal power and little to offer the manufacturer in terms of added value. True, the pharmacist was "the final link–the end-of-the-line–in what [was] essentially a marketing system for prescription drug manufacturers" (27). Nevertheless, the pharmacist was a channel member whose activities could be coordinated through authoritative control mechanisms and appeals to the power of the manufacturer.

CHANGES IN THE PRACTICE OF PHARMACY: ALTERING THE ROLE OF THE COMMUNITY PHARMACIST AND PHARMACEUTICAL MARKETING ACTIVITIES

Beginning in the 1970's, several changes in the environment began to broaden the scope of pharmacists' duties and subsequently their role in the selection and use of pharmaceutical products. Two of the most prominent changes were the growing roles of the pharmacist in generic substitution and in OTC drug product selection. As described in another article in this collection, leaders of organized pharmacy began working through state legislators in the mid-1970's to repeal pharmacy antisubstitution laws, leading to generic substitution in all 50 states (28). A pharmaceutical executive, Irwin Lerner of Hoffman-La Roche, commented that "the concept of substitution could, and probably already has, altered the nature of our business by superimposing the pharmacist's choice of drug product over the physician's" (29). The role of the pharmacist with respect to OTC drug product selection has also changed. Since the early 1970's, a number of active ingredients have made the switch from prescription to OTC status. The pharmacist can have a great deal of influence in a patient's selection of a drug product, and in some cases may actually serve as a substitute for a physician's visit and subsequent prescription drug purchase. Certainly the stature of the community pharmacist is enhanced by such activity (5).

These two changes in the environment forced pharmaceutical companies to rethink their message to and involvement with pharmacists. Lillian noted that:

> Before the repeal of anti-substitution, marketing executives regarded the pharmacist as a receptacle for their product lines: 'Ship it into the pharmacy and get the doctor to write prescriptions. The pharmacist has no choice but to stock the drug' . . . things are different now . . . more and more pharmaceutical manufacturers have realized that using the pharmacist as a consultant can not only increase the sale of the products, but also the relative importance of the company's lines. (30)

These changes, especially the issue of generic substitution, led to an increased emphasis being placed on advertising directed to pharmacists (31). Others encouraged manufacturers to get to know pharmacists better because of their increased role in the care of patients. Smith remarked that "in order for pharmaceutical marketers to realize the fullest potential of the partnership between manufacturer and pharmacists will require a much better understanding of the pharmacist by those who market to him and through him" (32).

While generic substitution and the increasing role of the pharmacist in OTC drug product selection have had profound effects on the practice of pharmacy and have forced pharmaceutical manufacturers to rethink their view of the role of the pharmacist, other changes in the environment have occurred over the past 30 years that have also greatly influenced the role of the pharmacy practitioner in the health care system. The nature and scope of pharmacy practice has received a considerable amount of attention, beginning in the mid-1960's with the birth of clinical pharmacy practice. The clinical pharmacy movement brought with it new pharmaceutical services, such as clinical pharmacokinetics, participation in patient care rounds, and drug information centers. Pharmacists were becoming more involved in drug selection beyond merely substituting generics for brand-name products.

Coinciding with the clinical pharmacy movement in the hospital environment was the growth and further development of pharmacy and therapeutics (P & T) committees and hospital formularies. This growth led to further expansion of the duties and responsibilities of the pharmacist. The role of the pharmacist in this setting was more than merely enforcing formulary decisions. After examining the influence of the pharmacist in affecting change in medication therapy above and beyond formulary maintenance in the hospital setting, Lazarus and Smith observed that "pharmaceutical marketers who feel their job is done when their product is on the formulary and the physician has written the order for it may be in for some surprises" (33). Changes in the nature and scope of pharmacy practice led Zellmer to encourage the pharmaceutical industry "to learn about the growing clinical movement in hospital pharmacy and to understand the ways practitioners in this field influence the use of drugs" (34).

Although the major concepts and innovations of clinical pharmacy came from institutional settings rather than from community practitioners, the clinical pharmacy movement had a substantial impact on pharmacy in general. For example, to encourage the development of a patient-oriented, clinical practice of pharmacy and to encourage pharmacists to use their professional knowledge, the American Pharmaceutical Association adopted a new code of ethics in 1969, removing language from previous codes that restricted the role of the pharmacist by prohibiting pharmacists from discussing the "therapeutic effects or composition of a prescription with a patient."

Despite its beneficial effects on pharmacy practice, the clinical pharmacy movement was still unable to completely move pharmacy away from the "count and pour" era of pharmacy practice (35). The practice of pharmacy in general continued "to focus on the drug and its delivery to abstract biological systems rather than to individual patients" (36). Community pharmacy, for the most part, continued to explore more efficient ways to dispense prescription products. As the realization was being made that the clinical pharmacy movement was more than likely going to be unable to dramatically effect change in pharmacy practice, especially in the community pharmacy setting, the profession began to recognize two other important points in the mid-1980's: (1) the practice of pharmacy was still in search of a professional mandate and (2) preventable drug-related morbidity and mortality was a prevalent and costly problem in medical care that could be addressed by pharmacy practice (36). It has been suggested that the mandate of pharmacy is "to help the patient obtain the best possible drug therapy and especially to protect the patient from harm," and this mandate is justified by the literature on preventable drug-related morbidity and mortality and the potential of pharmacy to prevent it (36). The mission of pharmacy practice, consistent with this mandate, is to provide pharmaceutical care, or "the responsible provision of drug therapy for the purpose of achieving definite outcomes that improve a patient's quality of life" (36).

The pharmaceutical care movement calls for a greater role of the pharmacist in the care of patients. It requires that pharmacists take responsibility for patient outcomes. The pharmacist "becomes the linchpin in achieving positive outcomes for the patient–intervening with physicians to assure proper prescribing and intervening with the patient to assure compliance and positive outcomes" (37). The role of the pharmacist is expanding. Although Adamcik and Rhodes make the following comment about pharmacist interaction with the elderly population, it is applicable to the population in general: "with good communication skills, pharmacists can obtain accurate medication histories, improve patient compliance, decrease the possibility of adverse drug reactions and interactions, prevent duplication of medications, simplify drug therapies, ensure cost-effective pharmaceutical care, and counsel elderly on all aspects of their drug therapy" (38).

The growing role of the pharmacist has been recognized by our legal system, where the "pharmacy profession is experiencing an increase in the legal responsibility resulting from incorrect or inadequate professional advice" (39). All states have altered their pharmacy practice acts or board of pharmacy rules to reflect drug utilization review and patient counseling mandates required by the Omnibus Budget Reconciliation Act of 1990. Several states have adopted regulations allowing pharmacists to initiate and modify therapy under protocol with a physician. Still other states have passed legislation allowing pharmacists to administer immunizations. The growth of managed care and disease management have also created opportunities for the pharmacist. The disease management model "provides the opportunity for community pharmacists to have a significant impact on the overall management of the patient" (37). Bailit sees the role of the pharmacist in HMOs and PBMs as substantial and growing, stating that much of the influence of the pharmacist is and will be at the population level (40).

The collection of articles in this issue demonstrates the past, growing, and potential roles of the pharmacist in a number of different areas. It is necessary for the marketer of pharmaceuticals to understand the roles of the pharmacist with respect to drug selection, patient counseling and education, disease management, patient compliance, and quality of life assessment and monitoring, as these roles are all reflective of the growing influence of the pharmacist in the care of the patient (28, 41-44).

As Zellmer states, "the goals of pharmaceutical care are consistent with the interests of the pharmaceutical industry. Fundamentally, it is to a drug company's advantage if the decisions about the use of its products are tailored to the needs of individual patients" (45). The evolution of the practice of pharmacy has the potential for benefiting not only patients and the practice of pharmacy, but manufacturers as well. The growing role of the pharmacist and the subsequent focus on the appropriate and optimal use of drug therapy represent significant opportunities for the manufacturer to establish close relationships with practitioners and the profession as a whole. However, a number of events have occurred that have not only strained the current relationship between pharmacists and manufacturers but have also made the possibility of establishing such long-term, cooperative relationships more difficult.

Although there are examples of manufacturers embracing changes in the practice of pharmacy and there are still more examples of manufacturers accepting these changes and recognizing the need to alter some of their promotional activities, the pharmaceutical industry has typically offered opposition to the evolution of the practice of pharmacy. The Pharmaceutical Manufacturers Association, along with the American Medical Association, was strongly opposed to the repeal of antisubstitution laws, and some companies offered opposition in the 1970's when organized pharmacy was fighting for FDA recognition of the role of the pharmacist as a consultant on nonprescription drugs (27, 32). Smith, in 1974, remarked: "I believe that the pharmacist may not see the industry as his partner anymore, but rather as some sort of adversary" (32).

More recently, the Pharmaceutical Research and Manufacturers of America (PhRMA), in a statement on proposed revisions of the Pennsylvania pharmacy practice act, objected to "proposed revisions pertaining to the expansion of the definition of the practice of pharmacy, the establishment by pharmacists of protocols or collaborative care agreements with physicians and others with prescribing authority, the involvement of pharmacists in disease management, and the reimbursement of pharmacists for conducting drug regimen reviews and for disease management" (12). Certainly not all manufacturers are opposed to changes that are occurring in the practice of pharmacy. For example, one pharmaceutical company representative has commented that "the company has 'tried to take a partnership approach with pharmacists, including providing programs and information on pharmaceutical care to help pharmacists play a more critical role in working with patients' " (11).

In addition to manufacturer opposition to changes in the practice of pharmacy, several other issues have strained the relationship between pharmacists and pharmaceutical manufacturers. Drug pricing policies of manufacturers and the practice of vertical integration (i.e., the combination of pharmaceutical manufacturers with pharmacy benefits managers and mail-order businesses) have angered many community pharmacists (9, 10). Additionally, some partnerships between pharmaceutical manufacturers and managed care organizations have initiated disease management and drug therapy programs that do not include pharmacists (20).

Despite the difficulties in overcoming the strain in the relationship between pharmaceutical manufacturers and pharmacists, increased partnership between these channel members has the potential to provide benefits not only for manufacturers and pharmacists but also for patients. Hussar calls for "greater communication and collaboration and the development of a true partnership between practicing pharmacists and the pharmaceutical industry" (12). The following sections discuss possible ways in which pharmacists and manufacturers can establish relationships, benefits to be gained, and methods by which manufacturers can reach their pharmacist colleagues.

FOSTERING RELATIONSHIPS: WHAT CAN PHARMACEUTICAL MARKETERS DO AND WHAT CAN THEY EXPECT IN RETURN?

As Silverstein observed, "the winning companies will be those that have implemented customized value approaches with marketing strategies that focus on individual customer segments derived from a thorough understanding of the economic structure of disease and a systematized knowledge of their potential customers" (46). Perhaps the most basic procedure for establishing relationships with pharmacists and hence implementing a customized value approach is providing valuable, useful, and accurate information to pharmacists concerning products. To assure appropriate use, pharmacists must be knowledgeable about pharmaceutical products, including information on safety, efficacy, and pharmacoeconomic outcomes. The focus of the information provided to pharmacists should no longer focus solely on the commercial issues associated with the drug product. Pharmacists need as much, if not more, clinical information as is provided to prescribers. Pharmacists are in a position to assure patient satisfaction with drug products (9). As Bootman and Noel describe, "pharmacists review medications with patients to verify and strengthen their understanding of the medication, how and when to take it, its desired effects, and likely side effects. Pharmacist counseling emphasizes information vital to the patient's understanding of treatment–reinforcing physician advice that patients often forget–thus enhancing the likelihood of a positive outcome" (47). Certainly, the manufacturer benefits (as well as the patient and the pharmacist) if positive outcomes are achieved and patient satisfaction is enhanced.

Information provided to pharmacists about drug products should be objective and should be based on good science. Sutters notes that many pharmacists have a low opinion of promotional information because of cases of deception (48). Other authors have described the potential of promotional activities to create ethical dilemmas and to alter the objectivity of pharmacists in drug therapy decisions (49, 50). Zoloth calls for ethical guidelines for the relationships between pharmacists and the pharmaceutical industry (51). The provision of useful, accurate, unbiased information should help to alleviate these ethical concerns.

The provision of product-specific information can help the pharmacist help the patient achieve optimal drug therapy outcomes. Additionally, the pharmacist should be an active member of any program aimed at the final consumers of drug products. For example, "pharmaceutical companies that market chronic medications could assist pharmacists by helping them develop and implement–and perhaps could even subsidize–practical and effective refill reminder systems" (52). Pharmacists should also be involved in disease state management programs, such as offering patient education and training on asthma or diabetes. Again, by utilizing the expertise of the pharmacist in compliance programs and education programs, benefits accrue to manufacturers, pharmacists, and most importantly, patients.

Pharmaceutical manufacturers can also establish valuable relationships with pharmacists by supporting and offering continuing education and other educational programs and services. The Internet offers pharmaceutical companies opportunities to be collectors and disseminators of information while also providing a valuable service to the pharmacy community. One example of a company that has been able to use the Internet to provide educational and other services to the pharmacy community is Glaxo Wellcome, which has offered its HELIX (Healthcare Education Learning & Information Exchange) web site (http://www.helix.com/). Among other services, the HELIX web site offers continuing education programs (on-line exams and grading), access to MEDLINE®, information on national teleconferences for health care professionals, information on the Pathway Evaluation Program® (career pathways) from Glaxo Wellcome, professional association web sites and discussion forums, and links to selected health information and health care news sites.

As stated earlier, changes in the practice of pharmacy, especially pharmaceutical care, are consistent with the interests of the pharmaceutical industry (45). Helping patients obtain the best possible drug therapy is a goal of pharmacy practice and should be a goal of the pharmaceutical industry. Thus, the pharmaceutical industry should support efforts by pharmacists to become more involved in the care of patients, as these efforts are in the best interests of manufacturers, pharmacists, and patients. In a study from England, Sutters and Nathan explored ways in which patients, practitioners, and the pharmaceutical industry could all benefit if the industry were to promote greater clinical involvement between pharmacists and general practitioners (53). Results from their study show that 86% of pharmacists and almost half of the general practitioners wanted the industry to hold joint meetings with both professions. The pharmacists and the general practitioners both reported that the industry should promote the role of the pharmacist in monitoring and improving patient compliance, in adverse drug reaction monitoring, and in giving advice to patients for minor ailments. The authors conclude by stating that "the results of the survey indicate that pharmaceutical companies should begin to target community pharmacists in their marketing plans to promote their involvement in [certain] types of activities" (53).

In addition to the benefits received from helping pharmacists help patients achieve better drug therapy outcomes, pharmaceutical manufacturers can undertake other relationship establishing efforts that will provide them with additional benefits. For example, several companies have established pharmacy advisory committees, and Hussar recommends pharmaceutical manufacturers should have at least one pharmacist on their board of directors (12). Advisory committees can be useful in trying to determine the effect of company policy and initiatives on pharmacy, in determining the needs and wants of this customer segment, and in providing valuable information on product development. Zoloth criticized such advisory boards, stating that "while I would like to believe these appointments were based solely upon my intellect, I cannot help but feel they may have been based upon my perceived purchasing authority. These advisory board experiences were almost always at some expensive resort" (51). Advisory committees should be established and operated with the goal of forming a true relationship based on mutual trust and not focused solely on selling more product. Benefits will accrue after the establishment of the relationship. Furthermore, holding advisory committee meetings at extravagant sites is costly and unnecessary.

Pharmacists at the community pharmacy level can also provide value to the manufacturer in postmarketing surveillance. Pharmacists can monitor and report adverse drug reactions and can be in a "position to develop hypotheses [for further Phase IV research] based on specific observations of drug safety, efficacy, interactions, reactions, and effects on health status, cognitive function, and quality of life" (54). Certainly, pharmacies and pharmacists can be involved in the collection of data for a Phase IV study.

FOSTERING RELATIONSHIPS: HOW TO REACH PHARMACISTS

Several benefits can be realized by establishing cooperative relationships with pharmacists, and a number of opportunities exist for fostering relationships. However, to establish relationships, pharmaceutical manufacturers need to be able to reach pharmacists. What is the best method for contacting community pharmacists to provide information? What journals do they read? What professional meetings do they attend? What associations do they belong to? What type of drug therapy information do they find most useful? To address these questions, Summers et al. conducted a national study of community pharmacists (55). Although their findings are somewhat dated, they do provide some suggestions concerning the most appropriate methods for contacting pharmacists to establish relationships. Because the data are five years old, the impact of the Internet was not addressed in this study. As mentioned earlier, the Internet has the possibility of serving as a valuable tool for providing information and education services to community pharmacists. Additionally, the Internet may offer the opportunity to receive valuable feedback from practicing pharmacists.

Summers et al. found that continuing education programs and journal articles provide the most useful information to community pharmacists. The authors state that "the results indicate that the best way to communicate with community pharmacists is to have sales representatives provide them with printed CE programs, reprints of journal articles, and product literature" (55). As mentioned earlier, information provided to pharmacists about drug products should be objective and should be based on good science.

Four journals, *American Druggist*, *Pharmacy Times*, *Drug Topics*, and *U.S. Pharmacist*, were identified by more than 90% of the community pharmacists as those that they read to some degree (Table 1). A fifth journal, *American Pharmacy* (now known as the *Journal of the American Pharmaceutical Association*), was reported to be read by 65.5% of the community pharmacists. The authors conclude that "these results suggest that pharmaceutical marketers can be confident in their current use of these journals to disseminate sponsored research results and CE programs" (55). Grussing and Wilkins conducted a similar readership study and found that "respondents reported reading their state journals more frequently than national publications" (56). State pharmacy journals were not included in the Summers study.

Summers et al. also found that the only meeting that community pharmacists attended more than once (on average) in the previous five years was their state pharmacy association annual meeting (Table 2). These results are consistent with the finding that over 90% of the community pharmacists are members of the their state pharmacy association (55). No other organization was found to have a membership

REFERENCES

1. McFadden TC. Marketing research takes its rightful place. Pharm Exec 1995; 15(2):70-5.

2. Worthen DB. Who is the customer? J Pharm Market Manage 1994;8(4):7-23.

3. Gans JA. The need for guidelines in pharmaceutical promotion: a pharmacy perspective. J Pharm Market Manage 1992;7(1):147-55.

4. Swann JP. The evolution of the American pharmaceutical industry. Pharm History 1995;37(2):76-86.

5. Robbins J. Pharmacy affairs: making the marketing connection. Pharm Exec 1986;6(9):40-4.

6. Higby GJ. Evolution of pharmacy. In: Gennaro AR, Chase GD, Marderosian AD, et al., eds. Remington: the science and practice of pharmacy. 19th ed. Easton, PA: Mack Publishing, 1995:7-17.

7. Roberts KB, Smith MC. Critical incidents in pharmacist/detailman relations. Med Market Media 1975;10(3):26-31.

8. Smith MC. Marketing to the pharmacist: who are the pharmacists? Med Market Media 1981;16(3):8-12.

9. Summers KH, Szeinbach SL, Barnes JH. Pharmacists' perceptions of retail pharmacy's professional image: implications for pharmaceutical manufacturers. J Pharm Market Manage 1994;8(2):43-58.

10. Lipson DP, Basara LA. Community pharmacists' perceptions of the pharmaceutical industry: a drug company image study. J Pharm Market Manage 1996;11(1): 43-59.

11. Zoeller J. 1995 survey: pharmacists rate manufacturers. Am Drug 1995; 212(1):23-5.

12. Hussar DA. Is partnership possible between pharmacists and PhRMA? Pharm Today 1997;3(4):4-22.

13. Morgan RM, Hunt SD. The commitment-trust theory of relationship marketing. J Market 1994;58(July):20-38.

14. Pelton LE, Strutton D, Lumpkin JR. Marketing channels: a relationship management approach. Chicago: Richard D. Irwin, 1997.

15. Weitz BA, Jap SD. Relationship marketing and distribution channels. J Acad Market Sci 1995;23:305-20.

16. Nevin JR. Relationship marketing and distribution channels: exploring fundamental issues. J Acad Market Sci 1995;23:327-34.

17. Juttner U, Wehrli HP. Interactive system's value creation through relationship marketing. In: Stewart DW, Vilcassim NJ, eds. 1995 AMA Winter Educators' Proceedings. Chicago: American Marketing Association, 1995:16-23.

18. Doucette WR. Opportunities for strategic partnerships between drug wholesalers and pharmaceutical manufacturers. J Pharm Market Manage 1997;11(3):3-22.

19. Vitali L. Partners for the future? Wholesale Drugs Mag 1994;46(3):48.

20. Harris N. Pharmaceutical companies seek partners. Am Drug 1995;212(2): 16-9.

21. Scott L. Valued components of value-added programs. Pharm Exec 1996; 16(4):82-4.

22. Joel HW. The power of precision targeting. Pharm Exec 1996;16(4):64-74.

23. Sheth JN, Parvatiyar A. Relationship marketing in consumer markets: antecedents and consequences. J Acad Market Sci 1995;23:255-71.

24. Peterson RA. Relationship marketing and the consumer. J Acad Market Sci 1995;23:278-81.

25. Bagozzi RP. Reflections on relationship marketing in consumer markets. J Acad Market Sci 1995;23:272-7.

26. Smith MC. Pharmaceutical marketing: strategy and cases. New York: Haworth Press, 1991.

27. Apple WS. Pharmacy's lib. J Am Pharm Assoc 1971;NS11:528-33.

28. Banahan BF. Community pharmacists' influence on prescription durg choices. J Pharm Market Pract 1998;1(2):11-35.

29. Lerner I. Issues and prerogatives. Med Market Media 1977;12(5):36-46.

30. Lillian BJ. Pharmacist's role as a marketing consultant to manufacturers on increase. Am Drug 1981;183(1):55.

31. Fink JL. Marketing in a generic environment: a pharmacist's view. Med Market Media 1979;14(10):40-6.

32. Smith MC. Can you dispense with pharmacists? Med Market Media 1974; 9(6):28-31.

33. Lazarus H, Smith M. After the order is written: pharmacist interventions in hospital drug therapy. Med Market Media 1988;23(6):76-80.

34. Zellmer WA. Getting to know hospital pharmacists. Pharm Exec 1986;6(9): 46-52.

35. Higby GJ. From compounding to caring: an abridged history of American pharmacy. In: Knowlton CH, Penna RP, eds. Pharmaceutical care. New York: Chapman and Hall, 1996:18-45.

36. Hepler CD, Strand LM. Opportunities and responsibilities in pharmaceutical care. Am J Hosp Pharm 1990;47:533-43.

37. American Pharmaceutical Association. Opportunities for the community pharmacist in managed care. Washington, DC: American Pharmaceutical Association, 1994.

38. Adamcik BA, Rhodes RS. The pharmacist's role in rational drug therapy of the aged. Drugs Aging 1993;3:481-6.

39. Hall M, Honey W. The evolving legal responsibility of the pharmacist. J Pharm Market Manage 1994;8(2):27-41.

40. Bailit H. Impact of managed care on pharmacy practice and education. Am J Pharm Educ 1995;59:396-400.

41. Juergens JJ. Trends in patient counseling and education. J Pharm Market Pract 1998;1(2):117-129.

42. Martin RE. Pharmacists and disease management. J Pharm Market Pract 1998;1(2):61-80.

43. McCaffrey DJ III, Wilkin NE. Leveraging community pharmacy to improve patient compliance. J Pharm Market Pract 1998;1(2):37-60.

44. Murawski MM, Bentley JP. Pharmacists and quality of life assessment. J Pharm Market Pract 1998;1(2):81-115.

45. Zellmer WA. Rethinking hospital pharmaceutical marketing. Am J Health-Syst Pharm 1995;52:1590.

46. Silverstein MB. A new paradigm for Rx marketing value. Pharm Exec 1992; 12(4):56-64.

47. Bootman JL, Noel M. Sampling on the line: should the giveaway war come to an end? Pharm Exec 1995;15(3):86-90.

48. Sutters CA. Drug marketing–co-operation between industry and drug and therapeutics committees. Pharm J 1989;243:131-4.

49. Poirier TI, Giannetti V, Giudici RA. Pharmacists' and physicians' attitudes toward pharmaceutical marketing practices. Am J Hosp Pharm 1994;51:378-81.

50. Wightkin WT. Objectivity in drug therapy. Drug Intell Clin Pharm 1985;19:55.

51. Zoloth AM. The need for ethical guidelines for relationships between pharmacists and the pharmaceutical industry. Am J Hosp Pharm 1991;48:551-2.

52. Levy RA, Smith DL. Staying the course: refill reminders can boost sales. Pharm Exec 1989;9(9):74-8.

53. Sutters CA, Nathan A. Can the pharmaceutical industry promote collaboration between community pharmacists and general practitioners. Pharm J 1993;250: 546-9.

54. Mendelson MA. Drug-regimen review and postmarketing surveillance: research links to consultant pharmacy. Consult Pharm 1988;3:313-9.

55. Summers KH, Banahan BF, Juergens JP, Jernigan JM. Marketing to the pharmacists: where will your promotion dollar most effectively reach pharmacists? University, MS: Research Institute of Pharmaceutical Sciences, 1992.

56. Grussing PG, Wilkins SM. Member readership of state pharmaceutical association journals. J Pharm Market Manage 1991;5(3):79-96.

Index

T - #0578 - 101024 - C0 - 229/152/9 - PB - 9780789010094 - Gloss Lamination